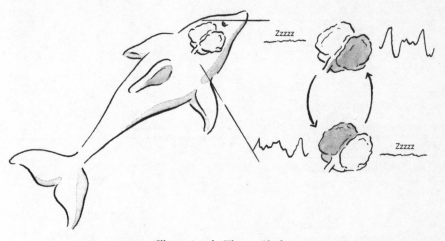

Zzzzz

Zzzzz

Illustrations by Thomas Shafee

the secret

world

of sleep

THE SURPRISING SCIENCE
OF THE MIND AT REST

PENELOPE A. LEWIS

palgrave
macmillan

THE SECRET WORLD OF SLEEP
Copyright © Penelope A. Lewis, 2013.
All rights reserved.

First published in 2013 by PALGRAVE MACMILLAN® in the United States—a division of St. Martin's Press LLC, 175 Fifth Avenue, New York, NY 10010.

Where this book is distributed in the UK, Europe and the rest of the world, this is by Palgrave Macmillan, a division of Macmillan Publishers Limited, registered in England, company number 785998, of Houndmills, Basingstoke, Hampshire RG21 6XS.

Palgrave Macmillan is the global academic imprint of the above companies and has companies and representatives throughout the world.

Palgrave® and Macmillan® are registered trademarks in the United States, the United Kingdom, Europe and other countries.

ISBN 978-0-230-10759-5

Library of Congress Cataloging-in-Publication Data

Lewis, Penelope A.
   The secret world of sleep : the surprising science of the mind at rest / Penelope A. Lewis.
      pages   cm
   Includes bibliographical references.
   1. Sleep. 2. Sleep—Physiological aspects. 3. Brain—Physiology. 4. Consciousness. I. Title.
QP425.L492   2013
612.8'21—dc23

2013019000

A catalogue record of the book is available from the British Library.

Design by Letra Libre, Inc.

First edition: August 2013

10 9 8 7 6 5 4 3 2 1

Printed in the United States of America.

contents

acknowledgments

I'D LIKE TO THANK ALL OF THE COL-leagues who have kindly helped with the research and fact-checking for this book, including Gorana Pobric and Patti Adank for the basics of the nervous system and brain anatomy; Simon Kyle for sleep physiology; Sue Llwellyn and Mark Blagrove for dreams; Jim Horne for the ubiquity of sleep and impacts of sleep deprivation; Rebecca Elliott and Deborah Talmi for emotion and emotional memory; and Dave Jones for the guerrilla guide to getting enough sleep. Special thanks also goes to Isabel Hutchinson for proofreading the entire manuscript and making many useful suggestions. Thanks also to my parents for their continual support and for their tireless proofreading and grammar-checking.

one

why sleep?

DO AMOEBAS SLEEP? THERE ARE CER- tainly times when they ball up and become inactive, but the true answer to this question depends on how you define sleep—and it turns out that there's more than one way to do that.

Using minimalist criteria, sleep can be thought of as an inactive time during which an organism responds less than usual when poked or disturbed, but from which it can be roused if danger threatens. This inactivity seems to have a purpose, since animals that are disturbed during such sleep invariably try to make up for it later on (we call this rebound sleep). Under this loose definition, amoebas actually *do* sleep. They stop moving, ball up, and become unresponsive even when prodded. They do this for hours at a time, normally at night, and they exhibit rebound if kept on the move and deprived of this restful state.

Insects, fish, and amphibians also sleep. In fact, every member of the animal kingdom appears to snooze at one point or another. In the case of wasps and others with antennae, this is particularly obvious since these appendages tend to droop when they snooze, signaling relaxed inattention to the environment.

Is sleep just something animals do when there are no demands on their time? Quite the reverse: Sleep is often a risky business. Most animals live in a predatory environment in which they are extremely vulnerable when they are not alert to surrounding danger. Many creatures could easily end up as a tasty snack if a predator manages to sneak up on them without being detected. This isn't only true for tender little critters like mice, parakeets, and tadpoles. Giraffes, for instance, take about 15 seconds to get to their feet after lying down for a snooze, so they are out of luck if a hungry lion happens to be in the area (it is probably for this reason that giraffes mainly sleep standing up or leaning against a tree, yet they also need to lie down for a short time every night to get some high-quality zzzzs).[1] Perilous as it is to snooze, it seems that sleep is so necessary that, like giraffes, other animals simply have to take the risk. Some, such as the parrot fish, which lives in wide open waters, have evolved clever strategies to limit the danger of catching forty winks. The parrot fish does this by creating a slimy, foul-tasting envelope around itself in order to deter predators who might otherwise have thought it would make a tasty nibble. Bottle-nosed dolphins and many species of birds and ducks have developed "split-brain" sleep, in which the brain activity patterns which indicate it is snoozing are limited to one side of the brain (called a hemisphere) at a time. The other hemisphere stays awake and controls an eye which keeps watch for dangers and also orchestrates some basic movements like swimming or using a flipper to stay afloat.[2] Split brain sleep poses an interesting question regarding consciousness: Is an animal truly awake or aware when only one hemisphere is active?

FUNCTIONS OF SLEEP

So what is the purpose of sleep? Surely something which is so widespread across the animal kingdom yet so dangerous and time-consuming must serve an important function. Alan Rechtschaffen, an important player in the history of sleep research, once said, "If sleep does not serve an absolutely vital function then it is the biggest mistake the evolutionary process has ever made."[3] As this statement suggests, scientists are reasonably unified in agreeing that sleep must be important, but ideas about *why* it is important vary hugely. One popular suggestion is that snoozing is a way to save energy. After all, animals don't normally move around a lot while they are asleep (unless we are talking about dolphins or other split-brain sleepers), so this state of inactivity must surely save some energy. This is a tempting hypothesis. We know, for instance, that many animals hibernate in order to save energy and hibernation shares many superficial characteristics with sleep—but hibernation typically lasts for months at a time, and body temperatures fall much lower during such periods than during sleep (sometimes to just a few degrees above freezing). Many animals actually warm up during hibernation in order to obtain a proper snooze. This means they are investing energy in order to get some sleep—suggesting that such slumber can't exist simply to make energy savings.

Another way to try and work out why sleep is important is by seeing what happens when we don't get enough of it. Sleep deprivation has been studied in great depth—from crude protocols in rats, who have been deprived of sleep to the point of death in many cruel experiments, to more carefully controlled experimentation on humans, whose brains, hormonal profiles, and ability to attend, remember, and make decisions have all been carefully analyzed after more limited periods of deprivation.

In one classic experiment, rats were housed on top of upside-down flowerpots in the middle of a pool of water. The flowerpot platform was above the water but small enough that the rats fell off it (and got wet!) whenever their muscles went limp (Fig. 1). Since one stage of sleep (REM, or rapid eye movement sleep) is characterized by total limpness of bodily muscles, this effectively meant the rats had a nasty wet awakening every time they reached this sleep stage. Rats who were treated in this way soon lost control of their body temperature, lost weight, and developed skin lesions. Within a few weeks they were all dead. This study suggests that sleep is important for temperature regulation and health in general (i.e., lack of deep sleep eventually leads to death), but it has been heavily criticized due to the excessive stress these rats suffered.[4] As you'd imagine, some of the criticism related simply to the cruelty of this procedure, which would have a hard time getting the approval of any contemporary ethics committee, but some of the criticism is also scientific. If you think carefully about the experiment, you'll soon realize that it is difficult to know whether it was really sleep deprivation that led to the untimely demise of these unfortunate creatures, or if their health problems could instead be attributed to the intense stress of the situation.

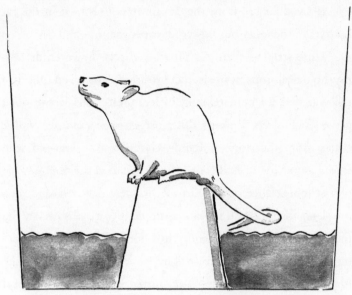

Fig. 1   Rat on top of inverted flowerpot

Subsequent experiments in rats have tried to answer this question, but none has completely satisfied the skeptics.[5]

Studies of sleep deprivation in humans have typically involved much less stressful situations in which, though deprived for long periods (sometimes 11 days or more!), participants are otherwise treated very carefully, know they can bow out of the experiment at any time if they really want to, and therefore have little real cause for anxiety. Nevertheless, these types of experiments have shown that sleep deprivation leads to an increase in the stress hormone cortisol, a small drop in body temperature, and compromised immune function. This suggests that, at the physical level, sleep plays a role in the maintenance of body temperature and immune response. Although not negligible, these effects are a far cry from the drastic responses seen in the rat martyrs of the infamous flowerpot experiment.

More striking than the physical effects, however, are the psychological impacts of sleep deprivation. There is no need to tell you that we humans tend to feel pretty lousy if we don't get enough sleep. Perhaps the most extreme example of this comes from the story of Randy Gardner, a 17-year-old who stayed awake for 11 nights in 1965 (a record at the time) as part of a school science project. In the first few days, Gardner had problems focusing and repeating simple tongue twisters. By the fourth day he showed memory loss and had minor hallucinations (e.g., imagining a street light was a person). After a week his speech had become slow and slurred, and by days nine and ten he had more marked cognitive impairments—for instance, when counting back from 100 he stopped at 65, apparently because he couldn't remember what he was doing. He also showed signs of paranoia, and his speech was slow and without intonation. However, Gardner's movement-based skills did not seem to be impaired. He won a game of pinball against a non-sleep-deprived interviewer on the tenth day of his ordeal. Although he had lost about 90 hours of sleep, Gardner only made up about 11 by oversleeping after the experiment, and he showed no evidence of long-term ill effects (though he was not, perhaps, monitored as thoroughly as he would be if such an experiment were to be conducted today, and I would certainly not recommend that any readers try this for themselves).[6]

Gardner's story serves to illustrate many of the impacts of sleep deprivation which have been shown by more carefully controlled and scientific experiments in larger groups. Namely, sleep deprivation can lead to moodiness, hallucinations, paranoia, poor memory, difficulty concentrating, and impaired decision making. These functions are all controlled by the brain, so this pattern suggests that sleep, or lack of it, impacts brain function even more than it impacts the body. This shouldn't come as a surprise, really, given that the brain orchestrates sleep and—far from switching off—moves through a complex and highly structured pattern of activities while you slumber. Let's take a closer look.

THE BRAIN IN SLEEP

We know the brain is active during sleep because scientists have spent a lot of time measuring this activity. The most common way to do this is by sticking little pieces of highly conductive metal onto the scalp. These electrodes can detect tiny electrical signals created by nearby brain cells (Fig. 2a). When you're awake, these signals show diminutive but continuously changing responses which can be used as a window on what's going on in there. For instance, electrodes show responses in visual areas of the brain when you see things, responses in auditory areas when you hear sounds, and so on.

While you're awake, there's plenty going on in your brain, so the overall pattern is of lots of small fast responses, and the electrodes produce what looks like a rapidly oscillating wiggly line (Fig. 2b). This is thought to reflect the fact that many of the different signals in there are going in different directions at the same time, so when they are added up they tend to cancel each other out. Picture the ripples in a small lake where ten speedboats are racing around, all going in different directions, and sometimes

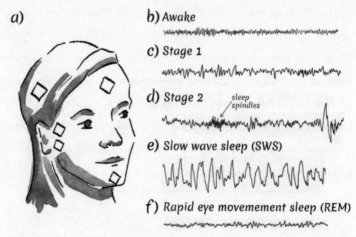

a)

b) Awake

c) Stage 1

d) Stage 2   sleep
                  spindles

e) Slow wave sleep (SWS)

f) Rapid eye movemement sleep (REM)

Fig. 2   *Example electrode placement (a), EEG during wake (b), increasingly
deep non-REM: stage 1 (c), stage 2 (d), slow wave sleep (e), and REM sleep (f).*

narrowly missing each other—these would be much messier than
the bow waves produced by a single boat going in one direction. As you get drowsy and start to close your eyes, the electrical signals from your brain slow down and get slightly bigger.
This slowing becomes more noticeable as you fall asleep—take
away a few speedboats so there is less interference, and imagine that the remaining boats get bigger, so they make slightly
larger waves (fig. 2c). We can tell when your sleep gets deeper
because new types of electrical activity called sleep spindles soon
start to appear on our electrodes. These are little bursts of frenetic
activity, often stemming from specific areas in the brain. Imagine now that children have started to jump off the remaining
speedboats into your lake, and each time they jump, they thrash
around in the water for a few moments before being scooped up
again (Fig. 2d). As you go still deeper into sleep the process of removing speedboats progresses, and eventually (when all of those

interfering bow waves start to settle down) you start to notice some huge rollers developing, almost as though the Loch Ness Monster is stirring up the depths, heaving itself up and down slowly and regularly at one end of the lake. It isn't just that you didn't notice these rollers before—they weren't there. These slow, high-amplitude waves are characteristic of deep sleep (Fig. 2e). They are a sign that, instead of doing lots of very separate tasks (as when disrupted by the speedboats), many areas of the brain are acting together in a coordinated, but slow, fashion.

All the steps I've described so far fall under the general category of non-REM sleep and can be divided into formal sleep stages. The stage when you initially fall asleep (just losing a few speedboats and slowing things down) is called Stage 1 non-REM. The stage when you lose a few more speedboats and the brain activity looks as though children have started to jump in and thrash around in various parts of the lake is called Stage 2 non-REM. The stage when you start to notice a lot of huge monster-induced rollers is called slow wave sleep—sometimes abbreviated SWS—thus named because of the slow movement of these high-amplitude rollers.

Importantly, the brain doesn't just move through these 4 stages of sleep once in a night. It cycles through them repetitively, with each cycle lasting about 90 minutes. Also, the time spent in REM and slow wave sleep is inversely proportional. You get a lot of slow wave sleep and little REM during the first part of the night, and show the reverse pattern later in the night. This means that if REM occurs at all in the first few 90-minute sleep cycles it is very brief—and the same is true of slow wave sleep during the last couple of cycles, when REM dominates.

All of this can be measured with electrodes on the scalp. And it turns out that, although your pulse and body temperature drop somewhat during the deeper stages of non-REM, there aren't too many other changes so far as your body is concerned. But what about rapid eye movement sleep (often called REM)? This sleep stage typically follows slow wave sleep, and although it is very deep sleep (and is indeed the time when we have our most emotional and bizarre dreams), what happens in the brain at this time is somewhat surprising. Instead of carrying on with the deep rolling waves, the sea monster who was generating them seems to calm down, and we instead see a return of the speedboats—almost as many as were there before you fell asleep. To speak more plainly, during REM sleep the electrical activity in your brain resembles the activity we see during drowsy wakefulness, in which it resembles the ripples in a lake with five or six large speedboats which aren't quite moving at full throttle (Fig. 2f). But this isn't the end of the story. The reason REM is named "rapid eye movement" sleep is because your eyes make rapid darting movements, usually under closed lids, during this phase. The eyes are the only area of the body where movement is possible, since all other skeletal muscles are paralyzed (which is why those poor rats kept falling off their flowerpots whenever they got into REM sleep).

How could this complex dance of sleep stages impact memory, mood, and decision making, and why should sleep deprivation lead to a meltdown in some of these systems? I will address all of these questions in later chapters, but for now let's just take a closer look at how sleep impacts memory.

SLEEP AND MEMORY

We know Randy Gardner had trouble with his memory after days of sleep deprivation, so losing sleep clearly has a negative impact upon memory. Related to that, there is a large literature of scientific studies which document cases when memory improves after sleep. The best examples are things like playing the piano or riding a bicycle: movement-based skills which don't require a lot of thought, and which we learn to do without necessarily being able to explain how we do them. These skills improve over a night of sleep, and the change can be dramatic.

A good example comes from a (pianolike) finger-tapping task in which people had to make a particular sequence of button presses as many times as possible in a minute. If you imagine numbering your fingers from pinky to forefinger (Fig. 3),

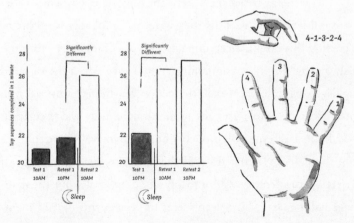

Fig. 3   The 4–1–3–2–4 sequence was tapped faster after a night of sleep

with one button per finger, the sequence people had to press was 4–1–3–2–4. When people practiced this during the day they got faster and faster until they eventually plateaued. Performance didn't change much if they were tested 12 hours later after staying awake all day, but if those 12 hours included a night of sleep, most people were much faster, tapping out up to 20 percent more sequences in a minute than they had done the night before.[7]

Matt Walker, the careful Berkeley scientist who did this experiment, first thought the lack of improvement across the day might be due to the fact that we use our hands (and fingers) to do all kinds of complex tasks; these activities might somehow have interfered with memory of the 4–1–3–2–4 sequence. He checked this by asking people to wear mittens during the day between test sessions. This had no effect whatsoever on the result, so the interference hypothesis went out the window. Instead, it looks as though sleep plays an active role in strengthening this type of memory.

Movement-based skills aren't the only types of memory that are influenced by sleep (if they were, you probably wouldn't be reading this book). Sleep impacts all types of memory—but not always by simply strengthening it. If I give you a list of word pairs to learn, e.g., cat-ball, tree-fence, bin-hit, etc., and ask you to repeat the whole list back to me straight away and then again 12 hours later, you will probably find that you've forgotten some of the pairs over that time. If the 12 hours include a night of sleep, your memory will probably *still* deteriorate, but the damage will be less. Thus, sleep seems to protect this type of memory, somehow preventing it from decaying as quickly as it would if the same period of time were spent awake.

The idea that sleep may simply prevent the pernicious effects of daytime interference holds a bit more weight in the case of word pairs than it did in finger tapping. Studies in which people have been kept inactive in bed without reading, talking, or watching films show that such sleepless repose can lead to a similar level of protection.

Nevertheless, those of us who study sleep and memory suspect there is more going on here than a simple absence of interference. After all, memory is a complex thing. In real life it is rare that we simply want to remember lists of word pairs. Most of the time we use our memories in a much more integrative way; we have a general knowledge of concepts, or frameworks of ideas, and we use these to dredge up individual facts which associate with these frameworks. For instance, we know what a birthday party is, and that it normally involves cake. We might also know what beetroot is, and that one of our friends who had a birthday party last year really loves this purple vegetable. Taken together, these two bits of information might help us to remember that she had beetroot cake for her birthday. If we didn't have the basic knowledge about birthdays and beetroot, that particular fact about her cake would be meaningless and therefore unlikely to be retained. There is a steadily growing bank of evidence supporting the idea that sleep plays a role in creating this type of underlying knowledge and in integrating new experiences into it.

SUMMING UP

This introductory chapter defined sleep and explained how widespread it is in the animal kingdom. We have looked at brain function during sleep, taken a peek at the negative impacts of sleep deprivation, and considered the role of sleep in memory consolidation. Chapter 2 will continue the story by providing an in-depth look at the sleep-deprived brain and explaining why lack of sleep leads to dulled senses, impaired decision making, low mood, poor memory, and even an altered moral compass.

two

how do we know sleep is important for the brain?

WHEN WAS THE LAST TIME YOU missed a full night of sleep? Maybe you were studying for an exam. Maybe a small child or baby kept you awake. Maybe you were just anxious and couldn't sleep. Or maybe you're an insomniac, and this is a regular thing for you. How did you feel? Probably not that good. Nevertheless, were you able to get on with your life the next day?

In general, people find they can do most things relatively normally after a night of sleep deprivation, even if they don't feel especially happy to be doing them. Most sporting abilities are unimpaired, as are IQ tests, reading comprehension, and performance on tests of logical deduction and critical reasoning. Don't let this fool you, however. Sleep deprivation also leads to major (and often dangerous) deficits. These are most dramatic in everyday tasks like driving a car. Driving is actually a really good example of a situation in which you have to remain alert and attentive for long, uneventful periods while you wait for a situation that needs a reaction. Think about blasting down a straight road with no need to slow or turn until someone pulls out in front of you. Even a little tiredness can slow down your reaction, meaning you hit the brakes later than you'd have liked. More serious fatigue can lead to attention lapses that could mean you don't even see that car until much too late—sometimes with dire consequences.

In many ways, a sleep-deprived brain acts like a brain under the influence of alcohol. In a hand-eye coordination task, each hour you are awake sets you back as much as an extra 0.004 percent alcohol concentration in your blood. This means every five hours you spend awake is roughly equivalent to one standard alcoholic beverage in terms of how your brain will perform. After 20 hours awake your performance is as impaired as if you had exceeded the legal limit in the United States (0.08 percent blood alcohol). Research into the impacts of sleep deprivation on the brain is responsible for the rapidly increasing number of sleep-related warning signs on our motorways. Happily, however, sleep deprivation's negative impact on vigilance and attention can be completely counteracted by caffeine—coffee addicts rejoice!—so a good coping strategy is simply to have a double espresso and wait 20 minutes for it to take effect before you get back on the road.

Strangely, younger people seem to suffer more in this situation than older people, not because they get less sleep but because they don't deal with sleep loss as well. It seems like the more aged and sage among us may develop coping strategies that help protect us against these types of errors. This could be used as a powerful argument against granting driving licenses at an early age; however, the counterargument that those of us who are old enough to have developed these skills don't want to work as taxi drivers any longer than necessary seems to beat this most of the time.

It isn't just boring activities like driving that are disrupted when you are sleep deprived. Plenty of evidence suggests that your basic perceptions of the world are also subtly changed when you are overtired. For a start, people are worse at guessing what smells are (is this rose or lavender?) and less likely to notice sour tastes when they are sleep deprived. There are also subtle problems with hearing (people have trouble telling which of two tones came first) and vision (people seem to pay more attention to things in the right-hand visual field).

So what is it about sleep loss that causes these impairments? One way of getting to the bottom of this is by doing the same task when you are well rested and when you are very tired, and comparing the brain activity in these two states. Studies that have tried this show that the extent of responses in a network of brain regions used for maintaining attention (prefrontal cortex, thalamus, basal ganglia, and cerebellum, see Fig. 4) is dramatically reduced in the sleep-deprived brain. Importantly, there is a direct relationship between how much activity in these areas is reduced and how tired you feel, as well as the extent of your cognitive impairment. Overall, this suggests that the brain's system of registering the external world through the five senses is weakened because you aren't paying as much attention to these

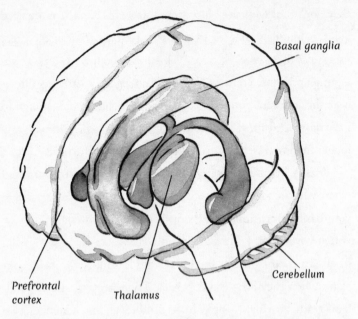

Fig. 4   Regions of the brain where activity is reduced in sleep deprivation

inputs when you haven't had enough sleep. The bias toward seeing things in the right visual field is associated with reduced activity in the visual processing areas of the brain, so this visual
impairment could also be due to altered attention.

When it comes to actual thought processes, it seems that
only the most complex tasks—those requiring creativity, lateral
thinking, innovation, and flexibility (for instance, the ability to
switch between two different rules, e.g., turn right or turn left in
order to get a reward)—are impaired by sleep deprivation. Sleep-
deprived people come up with fewer original ideas and also tend
to stick to old strategies that may not continue to be effective.
All of these processes rely on the front-most part of the brain, the

prefrontal cortex, so the fact that this brain region is less active than usual after sleep deprivation could partially explain these types of impairments. Surprisingly, high-level processes that require logical deduction, such as IQ tests and critical reasoning, are performed more or less normally even after two full nights without sleep. This finding suggests that such tasks don't actually rely on the prefrontal cortex as much as we previously thought.[1]

The sleep-related impairments of lateral thinking and flexibility seem to lead to some atypical decision processes. For instance, people tend to take more risks when they are sleep deprived. Studies of brain responses have suggested that, while such risk taking is associated with an abnormally strong response in areas of the brain that are active during rewarding experiences (like eating chocolate or having sex), the negative consequences that occur when things go awry (such as painful situations or those in which you lose something important) don't elicit the expected reaction in the brain's punishment system. Sleep deprivation also appears to impair moral judgments, by both slowing responses and increasing the chance that people will make choices that would violate their own moral position under normal conditions. All in all, this pattern suggests that the brain's system for punishment and reward is temporarily out of balance when people are sleep deprived. There is an interesting parallel between this imbalance and a similar pattern of activity observed in people who take bizarre risks on a daily basis (e.g., base jumpers, extreme skiers, and the like—see chapter 9).

Coffee may help you be more attentive and vigilant, but tiredness-related problems that involve mental and moral judgments are not alleviated by caffeine. This is not only bad news for the coffee dependent; it also suggests that these types of processes have a quite different neural basis from the types of deficits on which caffeine *does* have an impact, such as attention and vigilance.

On top of the problems mentioned so far, it will not surprise most people to hear that sleep deprivation distorts your emotions. Irrespective of how well you were able to get on with your day after that most recent night without sleep, it is unlikely that you felt especially upbeat and joyous about the world. Your more-negative-than-usual perspective will have resulted from a generalized low mood, which is a normal consequence of being overtired. More important than just the mood, this mind-set is often accompanied by decreases in willingness to think and act proactively, control impulses, feel positive about yourself, empathize with others, and generally use emotional intelligence. Sleep-deprived people are more easily frustrated, intolerant, unforgiving, uncaring, and self-absorbed than they would be if they were properly rested. All of these things combine to change the way they score on clinical mood disorder scales, often tipping perfectly normal people over the edge into the clinically relevant zone, so that, if tested on that particular day, they could be classified as depressed or even as psychopaths.[2] Although some of these problems may simply relate to low energy levels, evidence suggests that tiredness can also lead us to see the world through a negative filter. We are more likely to perceive perfectly neutral facial expressions as negative, and we are less able to appreciate humor. It isn't clear why all of this happens. One set of studies suggests that the specific region of the frontal lobe that usually filters negative feelings is impaired from lack of sleep. Therefore, the parts of our brain that respond to these negative perceptions (like the amygdala) get overexcited.

Students and parents of school-age children know from experience that sleep deprivation impairs learning. Neuroimaging studies have shown that the hippocampus, the part of the brain which is critical for learning new information, is markedly less active when you learn something after a night of sleep deprivation than when you learn the same information after a normal night of sleep.[3] This failure to engage the hippocampus translates into worse memory later on since the information you're trying to learn doesn't get properly engraved into your neural circuits. Interestingly, this temporary exhaustion-induced learning impairment doesn't seem to impact upon the retention of negative information. When sleep-deprived people were shown a list of words containing really unpleasant things (murder, rape, death), really nice things (beautiful, love, happy), and fairly neutral things (chair, plant, building), they were able to remember the negative words just as well as they would have if fully rested, but tended to forget the positive and neutral words.[4] It isn't really clear why this should happen, but we know negative information is often really important in the evolutionary context (you don't want to eat those poisonous berries a second time . . .), so it is possible that the extra resources are recruited to ensure this type of information is remembered even if you're dog tired. This suggestion has been backed up by brain-imaging data showing that a whole slew of additional brain regions are recruited if people learn about negative information (pictures in this case) while sleep deprived, and this isn't the case for neutral or positive information.

Although this extra emphasis on the negative may be good for avoiding nasty situations (and poisonous berries), it is actually a bit unfortunate from the psychological perspective since it means memories with negative content trump everything else. Combined with the negative filter through which tired people see the world, this could be the type of thing that puts people in a bad mood when they are sleep deprived.

SUMMING UP

This chapter has illustrated sleep's importance for the brain by showing that a whole range of mental processes are impaired if we don't get enough of it. Many brain areas are down-regulated when we are sleep deprived, and this means our senses are dulled, we lose creativity and lateral thinking, and our moral compass and decision-making abilities are altered. Sleep deprivation also disrupts new learning and leads to general low mood. These themes will be developed in more detail in future chapters; specifically, chapter 8 deals with the importance of sleep for lateral thinking and innovation, and chapters 9 and 10 deal with the impact of sleep on emotional processing.

three

building blocks of the brain

SUPERFICIALLY, YOUR BRAIN MAY appear to be just a pink-gray gelatinous mass, but it actually has a complex and highly regulated architecture. Cutting carefully into the jelly reveals multiple textures and shades. There is what we call gray matter, the cell bodies (or neurons), and white matter, the long, fat-coated connections between cells. The cell bodies can be thought of as the active processing agents of the brain, while the connections between them merely relay messages at the highest speed possible.

Looking more closely, possibly by slicing this unpromising pink-gray jelly in different directions, we soon find that both gray and white matter have different textures in different areas of the brain. This is because the microstructure, or the precise way in which cells are organized, as well as the precise types of cells present and the proportions of these types all vary between brain structures. In some areas, such as the large structure at the base of the brain called the cerebellum, cells are arranged in such a regular way that examination under a microscope reveals an almost crystalline regularity. In other areas, cells appear to be more haphazardly piled on top of each other. In most areas of the cortex, the densely folded covering on the top of the brain, cells are organized differently in each of several layers, with some layers receiving input while others seem more concerned with output. If awareness of these inputs and outputs makes you think of a computer, then you are right—the brain is just like a huge, complex computer in which the inputs, outputs, and the processing that occurs in between are all meticulously organized.

The gross anatomy of the brain—in terms of which regions and structures fulfill which functions—will be discussed

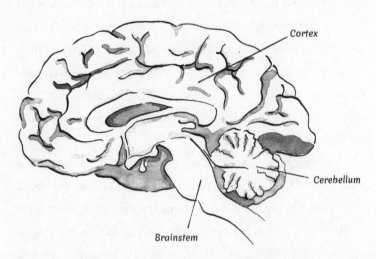

Fig. 5   Cross-section through the brain

in detail in chapter 6. In preparation for that (and for the rest of the book) we will use this chapter to take a close look at brain cells (or neurons), which are the building blocks of the mind, and explain how they use electrical charges to communicate and how subtle modifications in the way they interact provide the physical basis of memory.

BRAIN CELLS

So what are the fundamental units of this most gelatinous of all personal computers? There are many types of brain cells, but it is easiest to start out by thinking of them as having a fairly stereo-typed, cartoonlike structure (Fig. 6). The brain cell consists of a cell body, which contains the nucleus and most of the mass of the cell; a branching mass of dendrites (often called a dendritic tree), which receives inputs from other cells; and a long axon

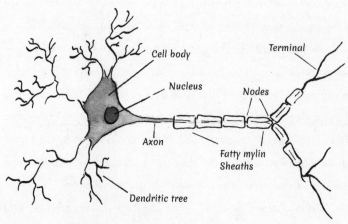

Fig. 6   Brain cell

that projects to other cells and potentially to other brain regions so a message can be relayed. It is these long, fat-wrapped axons that make up the white matter of the brain, while the less fatty cell bodies make up the gray matter.

To understand why nerve cells are special, we need to understand how they communicate, and that is determined by electrical charges both inside and outside the cell. The inside of a nerve cell has a negative electrical charge, largely because it is full of negatively charged proteins that cannot escape. On the other hand, the salty fluid outside the cell has a more positive charge. This is due to the presence of many positively charged particles such as sodium ions (Na+).

You will know from playing with magnets that polarity can lead to either repulsion or attraction. Particles with the same charge repel each other (positive repels positive and negative repels negative), while particles with opposing charges attract each other. This force, or electrostatic pressure, is present in the nerve cell since the inside has a negative charge and the outside has a positive charge. The difference between charges inside and outside the cell is called the membrane potential. The membrane potential acts both on the positively charged sodium ions, which would ideally like to move into the cell, and on the negatively charged proteins in the cell, which would ideally like to move out. The problem is that, while the cell is inactive, these particles cannot move because they cannot get through the cell membrane. However, the membrane is filled with tiny gates that are kept closed most of the time but can let these particles through when they are open.

When charged particles move through the membrane, and thus down the electrical gradient, they reduce the membrane potential. If this potential is reduced beyond a certain point, so-dium-selective gates open, and millions of sodium ions rush into the cell, further correcting the electrical imbalance. This quick change in the membrane potential is called an action potential. Action potentials allow nerve cells to communicate across long distances because the change in electrical potential at any given point on the cell membrane causes sodium gates at the next (neighboring) point on the membrane to open, and so the change in electrical balance propagates along the whole length of the cell.

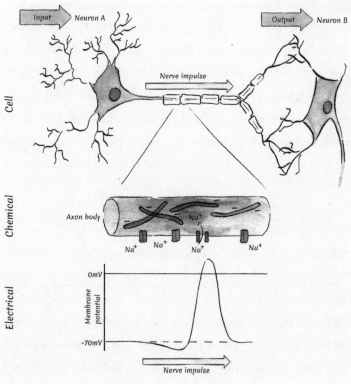

Fig. 7   The action potential

Axons are often tightly wrapped in fatty tissues that prevent ions from going in and out of the cell even when the membrane gates are open. When this happens, the ionic exchange can only happen at specific places (or nodes) on the axon that are not so tightly wrapped. This is important because it allows the action potentials to move along the cell very quickly, "jumping" from node to node.

Action potentials are very quick and transitory. This is because the rapid movement of ions across the membrane actually causes the inside of the cell to become slightly more positive than the outside. When this happens, the sodium gates close again, and they cannot be reopened until little pumps in the membrane have restored the original difference between sodium levels inside and outside of the cell. The action potential is over, and the cell is in an inactive, or refractory, period until the membrane potential has been returned to its original state. It may be this refractory period that causes us to talk about a cell "firing" action potentials—it takes a while to get the electrical gradient across the membrane set up, and once it has been rapidly changed (in an action potential), the cell can't fire again for a short time.

COMMUNICATION BETWEEN NEURONS

When neurons want to communicate one-on-one, they use something called a synapse, a place where the membranes of two different cells come very close together. The receiving side of the synapse is typically loaded with specialist receptors that can bind molecules that float across the synaptic cleft, while the transmitting side is loaded with little vesicles, or bubbles of membrane that encapsulate special chemicals (called neurotransmitters) that can bind to these receptors. When an electric impulse arrives at the transmitting side of the synapse, it triggers feverish activity in these vesicles—they bind to the cell membrane and release their contents into the fluid-filled void that is the synaptic cleft. The molecules of neurotransmitter that they were carrying then spread out in this fluid and quickly encounter the outer membrane of the target cell (on the other side of the synapse) with its hosts of receptors. The relationship between a neurotransmitter and a receptor is like that between a key and lock, but with the addition of electrical forces that bind them together in the right configuration. When a neurotransmitter touches an appropriate

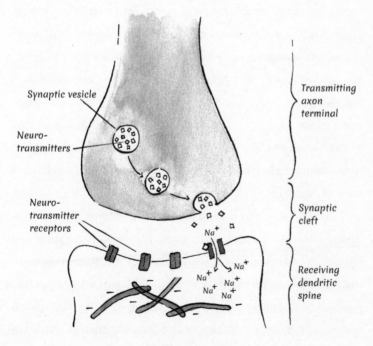

Fig. 8   The synapse

receptor, it is pulled in and becomes tightly fixed. This causes a cascade of activity in the surrounding cell membrane. If the neurotransmitter is *excitatory*, ion gates will open, sodium ions will most likely enter the cell, and this may eventually lead to an action potential. If it is *inhibitory*, it will cause the opposite reaction, increasing the difference between electrical charge inside and outside the cell, and thus decreasing the chance of an action potential.

Importantly, the binding of one or two neurotransmitters onto a cell is normally not enough to elicit a big reaction. The neurons onto which these chemical messengers bind can be thought of as integration machines: Most cells receive input from thousands of different sources but will only pass the message to other cells when this input is sufficient to trigger a strong, all-or-nothing action potential. The trick here is that not all of the inputs onto a given cell will have the same degree of influence. Some inputs may be very strong, and in extreme cases, a single synapse could even trigger the receiving cell to fire, while other inputs may be exceptionally weak, with thousands needed to elicit an equivalent response. Still other inputs can be inhibitory, counteracting the excitatory ones by moving the cell *away* from the state in which it might fire.

The way in which the cell constantly combines these various inputs and only becomes active when they sum up to a sufficient level of excitation means it is an incredibly sensitive integration machine. Couple this with the fact that the strength of various inputs can be altered over time, or by learning, and you may start to understand how the complex neural computer that is our brain actually works. Cells integrate information and pass on messages, but the importance of different types of input, and how likely it is to be passed on, can be altered according to the circumstances.

Indeed, this altering of the strength of various inputs is the physiological basis of memory. This makes more sense if you realize that different cells are carrying different types of information, so linkages between them can represent associations—for instance, between a face and a name or a candy bar wrapper and a chocolate taste. Of course, it takes more than just two neurons to build these memories, but the basic principle of strengthening a synapse extends to whole neural populations.

SYNAPTIC PLASTICITY

How can the strength of a particular input be altered? The receiving cell simply becomes more sensitive to these types of inputs. Metaphorically, we could compare it to the way you become more sensitive to verbal input from a friend if that friend suddenly becomes especially significant to you—for instance, if you suddenly find you are sexually attracted to him or her. In this case, inputs from your friend might become two or three times as important to you, and consequently two or three times as likely to cause you to act. At the same time, inputs from other people, such as your previous partner or less attractive friends, might lose salience and be less likely to cause you to act. The extent to which you respond to input from different friends is changeable or "plastic." If you were a neuron, we would call this type of flexibility "neuroplasticity," or an ability to alter how likely you are to respond to inputs from any given source. The metaphor only goes so far, of course, since cells neither have friends nor become romantically involved with each other.

So what makes one brain cell sit up and pay special attention to another? There is a little rhyme that answers this: "Neurons that fire together wire together." In other words, if a neuron becomes active and fires at the same time as it receives input from a particular source, the importance of information from that source will be strengthened in the future, and it will more likely cause the receiving neuron to fire. This could be likened to your tendency to listen more to friends who have given advice you acted on in the past. If a cell strengthens the impact of input from another cell, the connection between them is said to be "potentiated," or made stronger. Potentiation of this type can be transitory, but it can also be semipermanent. In the latter case, it is called long-term potentiation, and this type of long-term strengthening of connections is thought to form the neural basis of memory.

Let's take a closer look. Imagine you have ten friends, each of whom has an equal amount of influence on you. You need positive input from at least two friends in order to take action, so we could say you have a threshold of two. One day, a tricky decision comes up, and six of your friends give advice: four in favor of action and two against. Integrating these various inputs gives a net positive input of two—which passes your threshold, and so you act.

If you are a neuron, under the principle of "neurons that fire together wire together," we can now expect you to change the strength of your connections to these various friends (who represent other neurons). Specifically, you will strengthen the connection with the friends who advised you in favor of an action you chose to make, so these friends will have more influence on you in the future. In other words, you *remember* that you acted on the advice of these friends in the past, so you're predisposed to pay more attention to them in the future. As time goes by, and you experience the cycle of advice, action, and modifying a connection strength again and again, you may come to rely very heavily on specific friends, while others have almost no remaining influence. We would then say you have a very strong connection with those influential friends, or in terms of neurons, you have formed a very strong communication channel, or synapse.

One important constraint here is that, for neurons, connection strengths are generally only altered if the input (advice) and output (decision) are concurrent. Neurons cannot remember advice and then act on it a week later; they can only sum up the input present at any given moment, though this may linger for a few instants before disappearing completely (and remember, this input is actually made up of the influx or efflux of electrical charges, changing the overall electrical membrane potential). Moreover, if a neuron has a threshold of TWO for action, it must receive those two inputs at the same time, not sequentially. This means your friends would need to be providing information simultaneously, so speaking out loud might not be the best way to communicate.

In physiological terms, this means you would need excitatory neurotransmitters from two different input cells to contact your receptors at the same time. This would open up two sets of gates in your cell membrane, and would therefore let two lots of charged particles (probably sodium ions) flow in. If your threshold for action was TWO, then the movement of these sodium ions would change your membrane potential sufficiently to ensure you fired an action potential.

SUMMING UP

This is the most technical chapter of the book. It has explained the basic principles of how brain cells communicate and store information. We have introduced neurons as electrically charged entities and explained how the opening and closing of tiny, electrically sensitive gates in their membranes causes them to fire electrical action potentials. We have talked about how these changes in electrical potential can travel along neurons, and how neurons communicate by releasing neurotransmitters at synapses. Most importantly, we have introduced the idea that changes in one neuron's influence upon another, or synaptic plasticity, provides the physical basis of memory. All of this information is essential background for the rest of the book. In particular, chapter 4, which describes brain systems for sleep, draws heavily on the idea of neurotransmission, synapses, and action potentials.

four

how the brain controls sleep

POPPING A PILL OF ECSTASY IS A SURE-
fire way to get a rush. The response is strong and rapid since the
drug is absorbed quickly into your blood. But what does this
little tablet actually do to your brain? Why does it lead to such a
marked change in how you feel?

Psychoactive drugs work by disrupting the brain's natural
communication systems. This is true whether they are what
we'd call recreational drugs—as in the case of ecstasy, cocaine,
and marijuana—or clinical drugs such as those used to treat
depression, insomnia, anxiety, and schizophrenia. These chemical substances easily disrupt communication because the brain
uses chemicals as its basic messaging currency. It relies on the
movements of chemical messengers, otherwise known as neurotransmitters, which diffuse through extracellular spaces and

sometimes bind onto neurons, causing either excitation or inhibition. The process by which these chemicals are secreted in the right places, diffuse to the correct cells, and bind onto just the right targets is extremely delicate. Psychoactive drugs can disrupt it in lots of different ways, which means the messages your brain or body is trying to send get scrambled. For instance, they can mimic genuine neurotransmitters by clogging up the receptors where a specific neurotransmitter would normally bind, thus preventing the neurotransmitter from communicating its usual message. These drugs can also work by causing neurotransmitters to be released from storage, or by preventing those that have already been released from being recaptured and put back into storage at the normal rate, thus causing them to accumulate in abnormally high concentrations in the synaptic cleft.

Importantly, there are lots of different types of neurotransmitters, and they don't all do the same thing. Some lead to excitation, opening tiny channels in the membrane so that positively charged sodium ions rush into the cell and push it toward the threshold for firing an action potential, and some have the reverse effect, reducing the probability that a cell will fire. A neurotransmitter can only act on cells that have receptors which are specifically designed to fit it (remember the lock and key analogy). So even though a chemical may be sprayed throughout the whole brain, it will only act on specific types of cells in specific brain structures—and this means its action can be very targeted.

Just like people, brain cells sometimes communicate one-on-one, but sometimes they also need to broadcast their views to a large community. You know from chapter 3 that the one-on-one communication occurs at the synapse, where the outer membranes of two cells come very close together and neurotransmitters diffuse between them. When cells want to broadcast information to a wider audience, they tend to bypass the synapse. Neurotransmitters are released from other places on the cell, which allows them to reach much larger areas of the brain. The best analogy for this is broadcasting on a radio, as compared to phoning someone for a private conversation. When neurotransmitters are used in this way, we often call them neuromodulators because they influence the activity of whole populations of neurons by controlling their chemical state and can either dampen or heighten responses to other stimuli. Neuromodulators can stay around for long periods once released (up to 20 minutes) and can diffuse across large areas of the brain.

So how does all of this relate to sleep? If you have ever taken sleeping pills, you won't be at all surprised to hear that we fall asleep and wake up based on the actions of a complex cocktail of neurotransmitters. A summary of how some of the most frequently occurring neurotransmitters promote sleep and wake would go something like this: *Acetylcholine* is one of the most common neurotransmitters in the brain. It is essential for staying awake. This is the primary neurotransmitter of an arousal system that carries signals from the brainstem up to most of the rest of the brain. When this system is active it is constantly prodding the brain, knocking on the door, and saying, WAKE UP. *GABA,* on the other hand, is an inhibitory neurotransmitter. It tends to turn things off, or at least dampen responses. GABA is essential for sleep since it counteracts the alerting signal of the arousal system. This is particularly striking in animals such as dolphins, who sleep with just one hemisphere at a time. *Serotonin* is known

for its involvement in depression as well as for the way it interacts with recreational drugs like ecstasy (which indirectly boost
serotonin levels, leading to temporary feelings of euphoria).
When it comes to sleep, serotonin is essential because it inhibits
some of the actions of acetylcholine and can therefore cause you
to fall asleep. Paradoxically, however, serotonin can also promote
wakefulness under certain conditions, and concentrations of this
neurotransmitter are highest while you are awake.

That is the simple story of how chemicals control our sleep,
but of course reality is a lot more complex. Lots more neurotransmitters get involved, and there are different cocktails of
transmitters for different sleep stages. In order to explain this
in a bit more depth, let's consider a couple of early pathologies
that led to an initial understanding of how sleep and wake are
regulated in the brain.

BRAIN SYSTEMS FOR SLEEP AND WAKE

In the 1920s a strange disease swept through North America and
Europe. People who caught it simply couldn't get enough sleep.
Many of them were dead to the world for 20 hours a day or
more, waking up only long enough to eat and go back to sleep. A
famous neurologist, Count von Economo of Vienna, studied the
phenomena and wrote, "Patients left to themselves fall asleep in
the act of sitting and standing, and even while walking, or during meals with food in the mouth. . . . If aroused, they wake up
quickly and completely, are oriented and fully conscious . . . but
soon drop back to sleep."[1]

Quite understandably, this disease was called the sleeping sickness, or Encephalitis lethargica (this is not to be confused with African trypanosomiasis, which is also often called sleeping sickness). Count von Economo studied the disease, and his investigations eventually revealed that the sleeping sickness was associated with severe inflammation of a brain area called the posterior hypothalamus. Because damage to this area led to such semicontinuous slumber, von Economo reasoned that it must be important for keeping the brain awake.

Subsequent work showed he was right. It turns out that wakefulness is initiated and maintained by the arousal system, a set of neural projections called the ascending reticular activating system (ARAS). This system consists of a collection of ganglia (clusters of neurons) in the brainstem that send strong WAKE UP signals to the rest of the brain, using acetylcholine as well as a host of other neurotransmitters (Fig. 9). These messages pass through the posterior hypothalamus region that was damaged in von Economo's sleeping sickness, which almost certainly explains why his patients had trouble waking up. In fact, experiments on rats show that damage to this region in our furry friends also results in continuous slumber.

Collectively, all of this tells us that the ARAS system is important for keeping the brain awake. Importantly, the ARAS system contains two separate pathways. In one, a collection of brainstem nuclei project directly to the cortex, providing a strong arousal signal. In the other, separate brainstem nuclei project to the thalamus, and thus promote the arrival of sensory information to the cortex, which acts as an alerting signal.

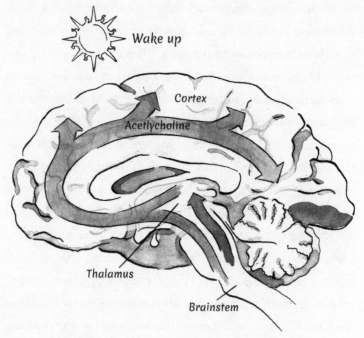

Wake up

Cortex

Acetlycholine

Thalamus

Brainstem

Fig. 9   Ascending reticular activating system (ARAS)

Interestingly, however, not all of von Economo's patients had trouble staying awake. Some of them had the exact opposite problem—severe insomnia. Through careful postmortem examination of the brains of these patients (some of whom eventually died of the disease), von Economo discovered these people had damage to a different brain region, the preoptic area. Because this damage led to problems falling asleep, he reasoned that this area must be critical for that side of the story, and again, he was right. More recent studies have shown that bilateral lesions to this region in rats lead to continuous wakefulness. So the preoptic area is critical for initiating and maintaining sleep.

Exactly how does the preoptic area perform its sleep-promoting function? The neurons in the preoptic area project downward toward the brainstem, where they communicate with the neurons of the ARAS (wake up) system and effectively shut them off, preventing the WAKE UP signal from reaching the rest of the brain and allowing you to fall asleep. Preoptic neurons also prevent cells in the brainstem from passing on information about sounds and other external stimuli that might wake you up. The neurons in this area are maximally active in non-REM sleep, less active in REM sleep, and minimally active in wake.

Communication between the preoptic sleep-promoting system and the ARAS wake-up system is not a one-way street. Neurons in the ARAS system project to the preoptic area and, given the chance, they can even shut *those* neurons off. So these two systems (wake-promoting ARAS and sleep-promoting preoptic area) are actually reciprocally interconnected; each one inhibits the other. Figure 10 shows how this works. You may notice whichever side is switched on most strongly will dominate and firmly keep the other side off. This is a core characteristic of sleep-wake regulation and helps to explain why we spend so little time in a semi-asleep phase. We're either sleeping or we're not—that's what this arrangement tries to ensure.

In engineering terms this arrangement would be called a "flip-flop" switch because it is only stable when you are in either wake or sleep—but not in the in-between phase. The balance of this switch is very slowly altered as you get tired and sleep pressure increases across the day, and also as circadian input gradually shifts to indicate that it is time to sleep. Both of these forces

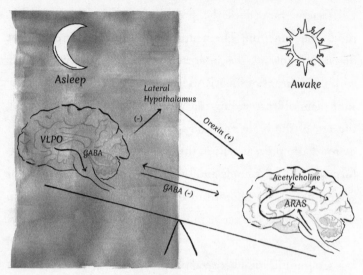

Fig. 10   The sleep/wake flip-flop

modulate the probability of a rapid transition between wake and sleep. You can think of the system as a kind of seesaw—it is most stable when one side is fully down and the other side is fully up (for instance, if you're awake). If a pressure (like sleepiness and/ or late time of day) presses on the up side and gradually pulls it down, the system will become increasingly unstable until it flips into its other stable state (sleep).

Of course, it isn't always a good idea to flip quickly between wake and sleep. In fact, there's a fairly nasty disease called narcolepsy in which the main problem is the tendency to do just this. A large proportion of people with narcolepsy fall asleep at the drop of a hat, and this is (quite counterintuitively) particularly likely if they are suddenly excited or frightened. People with narcolepsy not only fall asleep when driving or listening to a boring

lecture, they can also suddenly succumb when laughing, playing games with friends, running around, or telling jokes. The
sudden somnolence is especially striking because they don't just
fall into any sleep stage: They go straight to REM sleep, which
you'll remember is characterized by paralysis of bodily muscles.
A sudden transition from running around laughing to REM
sleep means not only sudden unconsciousness, but also physical
collapse. People with narcolepsy literally melt into a pile, as all
their bodily muscles relax when they enter REM.

Why does this happen? It turns out narcolepsy is caused
by abnormalities in a neurotransmitter called orexin. Orexin is
produced by the lateral hypothalamus and acts to stabilize the
sleep-wake flip-flop. By stimulating the ARAS system, this neurotransmitter helps to keep us awake, and thus biases the whole
system toward wake rather than sleep. When orexin is absent
or abnormal, the extra stability it normally provides is lost, and
the system is able to switch more easily into sleep (as we see in
people with narcolepsy).

Why do people with narcolepsy specifically fall into REM
sleep? Because orexin not only promotes wake, it also specifically inhibits a group of cells that promote REM (the "REM-on"
cells). So removing orexin means these REM-on cells are overactive, and people with damage to this system are always at the
point of dropping into REM. The REM-on cells are also excited
by the amygdala, which responds to scary situations—so these
highly arousing times are actually also the times when the REM-
on cells are most strongly active and most likely to take control.
Given this physiology, it should be clear why antidepressant drugs
(which block REM sleep) are the main treatment for narcolepsy.

Of course, narcolepsy isn't the only disorder of the sleep-wake system. Insomnia is one of the most commonly experienced disorders of sleep. Insomnia can be caused by either excessive activity in the arousal system (usually the hypothalamus and upper brainstem) or concurrent activation of both wake-promoting and sleep-promoting pathways. This latter situation explains why some people with insomnia report poor sleep in the absence of any obvious sleep abnormality.

NEUROCHEMISTRY OF SLEEP

In the healthy brain, neurotransmitters perform a complex dance as they lull us to sleep, move us through the four sleep stages, and then wake us up again. Systems like ARAS and the preoptic area communicate with the rest of the brain using neurotransmitters, which means brain concentrations of several such molecules change dramatically as we move through the various stages of consciousness. The most dramatic example of this comes from acetylcholine, the brain's primary WAKE UP signal. In REM, despite the fact that you are deeply asleep, the electrical activity in your brain looks pretty much the same as when you are awake; that's why we call REM paradoxical sleep. It turns out that acetylcholine is present in REM at an even higher concentration than it is during wake. To be precise, there is *twice* as much acetylcholine floating around the brain during REM as during wake. This is interesting because acetylcholine concentration drops to near zero during deep slow wave sleep. It looks as though the WAKE UP signal needs to be turned off before we can get into slow wave sleep, but it also needs to be switched on again—and twice as strongly—if our brains are to get into the paradoxically active state of REM. If high levels of acetylcholine are really critical for REM sleep, then anything that prevents this concentration from increasing should also prevent you from getting REM—and that is exactly what happens. Serotonin inhibits the action of acetylcholine, and imbalances of serotonin not only wreak havoc on mood and motivation, they also mess up your sleep patterns. Too much serotonin inhibits REM, while too little can lead you to spend excessive amounts of time in this sleep stage. You are probably aware that low levels of serotonin are linked to depression and anxiety. Low levels of this neurotransmitter are also linked to insomnia probably because the excessive REM people experience in this state means they don't get enough slow wave sleep, and therefore feel extremely tired. A common class of antidepressant drugs, the selective serotonin reuptake inhibitors (SSRIs), can help with some of these problems. These drugs boost serotonin levels by interfering with the molecules that cleanse it from the system after it has been released. This means serotonin hangs around longer, so the overall concentration is higher than it would otherwise have been. Such increased serotonin not only improves mood, it also reduces the total REM you obtain, potentially increasing the time available for slow wave sleep. Unfortunately, SSRIs also disturb sleep continuity and induce periodic limb movements, so they are certainly not a panacea for treating insomnia.

Incidentally, the neurochemistry of sleep isn't something we have to leave totally to its own devices. Serotonin levels can be raised by exercise, calming activities such as yoga, and eating foods that contain the building blocks for serotonin, such as chicken, fish, and soy products. You might not think much about such things, but when was the last time you drank a cup of coffee to feel more alert? Caffeine interferes with the normal dance of neurotransmitters that control sleep by blocking the receptors for adenosine, a by-product of energy use that accumulates during our daily exertions. Adenosine makes us feel tired, but if the receptors it binds to are clogged up by caffeine, it can't have this effect—which is why you feel so alert after that early morning cappuccino. Of course, you can also become tolerant to caffeine if you consistently have a lot of it, but no matter how tolerant you are, it still stays in your system for up to ten hours and causes your sleep to be significantly lighter. If you think your five daily espressos are having no impact at all, just try going without them for a week. The built-up dependence will probably lead your body to protest with skull-splitting headaches and cravings for coffee. It is probably best to resist these if you really care about your sleep!

What about alcohol? Many people (particularly shift workers) like to use alcohol as a way of getting to sleep. Alcohol reinforces the inhibitory signals of the GABA neurotransmitter and thus helps to switch off the arousing ARAS system, allowing you to drop into non-REM sleep. A swift tipple will definitely make you drowsy, but there are some serious catches. Aside from the fact that alcohol is highly addictive and generally bad for most bodily systems, there are also good sleep-related reasons for not falling into this habit. Alcohol-induced sleep may start out relatively well, but the initial happy slumber is usually followed by lots of waking up, more dreams than usual, and a high proportion of nightmares. Headaches and dry mouth can be added to this list for frequent abusers. Some of these problems are caused by the rapid metabolism of alcohol, since your body starts to suffer withdrawal symptoms after the first few hours. In a nutshell, alcohol intensifies sleep disorders rather than helping to sort them out. There's even a clinical diagnosis called alcohol-induced sleeping disorder, which is applied to people who consistently use alcohol (even in very small amounts) to get to sleep. Don't join them!

What does all this have to do with how sleep impacts upon memory? It is clear that neurotransmitters control the interactions between neurons, so the complex and ever-changing dance of these powerful little chemical compounds during sleep must have an impact upon the consolidation that occurs. The standard theory of consolidation states that newly learned information is initially coded in the hippocampus but will gradually become independent of this structure as gems of knowledge are transferred to the neocortex through a process of consolidation. Projections from the hippocampus to the neocortex are inhibited by acetylcholine. It has been proposed that the drastic reduction in this neurotransmitter during slow wave sleep is therefore essential to allow the transfer of knowledge between these two structures. An empirical test supported this by showing that the memory advantage which usually results from this sleep stage was completely abolished when acetylcholine was artificially maintained at high levels in slow wave sleep.

SUMMING UP

This chapter has pointed out how powerfully neurotransmitters and the chemicals that interfere with them can impact the brain. It explained that different neurotransmitters work in different ways and outlined the main chemical compounds which are used to control sleep and wakefulness. We took a look at Count von Economo's sleeping sickness and how this unlocked the secret of two competing systems: ARAS, the arousal system which projects from the brainstem up to the cortex shouting WAKE UP, and the preoptic area which inhibits ARAS in order to promote sleep. We also looked at some common disorders of the sleep wake system, including narcolepsy and insomnia, and some ways in which people can manipulate their own brain chemistry to be more alert, get better sleep, or just feel good. The next chapter takes a closer look at the marked physical changes that occur in the brain during sleep and explains how these are tightly linked to the idea of memory consolidation.

five

mental spring cleaning
while you sleep

IF YOU HAVE A GARAGE, ATTIC, OR
even a large space under your bed, you will know how easy it is
for this to turn into an accumulation zone for random objects.
You will also know that having lots of things stuffed away in
there isn't always a good idea. Sure, you may have saved every
yogurt container and rubber band that ever came your way, but
excessive clutter almost always means it will be harder to find
the things you really want when you want them. This general
principle of storage space is equally true for the brain: It is better to store just the most important things and throw out the
unwanted garbage. The usual way of making this happen is by
having a regular clean-up time when the critical stuff gets separated from the trash.

There is strong evidence that sleep, and specifically slow wave sleep, provides a sort of spring cleaning for the brain. It turns out there is a limit to how much synaptic connections between neurons can be strengthened. Think back to the parallel between how synaptic inputs control the response of a neuron and how advice from friends controls your decision making. If you wind up with five friends, each of whom has so much influence over you that you instantly follow their advice without attention to anyone else, your decision making may become noisy and suboptimal. In the same way, if you strengthen too many input synapses onto any given cell, further strengthening becomes almost meaningless, as the cell is already hyperstimulated. During a day of normal experience we encounter lots of information, most of which is useless and need not be remembered. Unfortunately, our brains don't always filter this information efficiently, and this means lots of synapses get strengthened, some relating to important information we want to remember, some relating to unimportant information, and some relating to the pure meaningless noise. This means that by the end of the day our synapses are a mess. Just as we sometimes feel exhausted after a lengthy period of stimulating activity with no chance to rest, the resource available at a synapse can also be exhausted. Synapses can be overpotentiated, meaning they've been strengthened to the point where they can get no stronger. They can also be saturated, meaning they are potentially unable to take in new information. They cannot function optimally in this state. Something has to happen in order to clean up the mess, reset the synapses, and get rid of the unwanted information that has been stored. That something is sleep.

An elegant theory, called the synaptic homeostasis model (Fig. 11), proposes that slow wave sleep resets the whole system by globally downscaling synapses (in other words, by gradually weakening or de-potentiating them).[1] This downscaling not only makes space for new learning, it also removes noise and (assuming the important information has been encoded more strongly than unimportant information) increases the ratio between that

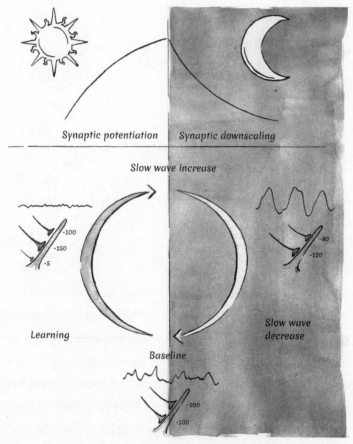

Fig. 11   The synaptic homeostasis hypothesis

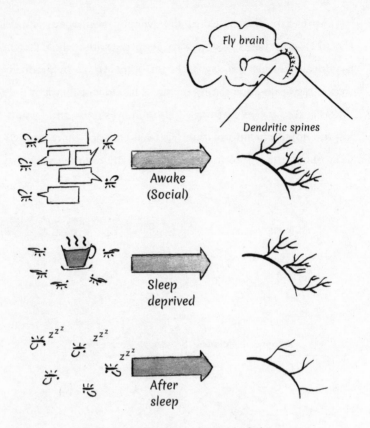

Fig. 12   *Synaptic homeostatis in the fly brain*

important information and noise. This can be compared to turning down the volume on a radio so that the background static can't be heard—even though the overall output is quieter it is still easier to understand what is being said once the noise has been removed.

The strongest support for synaptic homeostasis comes from studies conducted in the fruit fly *Drosophila melanogaster* by Ciara Cirelli, Giulio Tononi, and colleagues at the University of Wisconsin.[2] These researchers made a really clever choice by working with fruit flies since this allowed them to examine the physiological state of synapses after different wake and sleep experiences in a way that wouldn't be possible in the human brain. This rather invasive scrutiny showed that synapses grew in size and number during wake and decreased only when the flies were allowed to sleep. Fascinatingly, the extent of synaptic growth was determined by what each fly experienced during the day—so flies placed in a highly social environment (a fly mall, with lots of other flies) showed substantially more synaptic growth than flies kept in solitary confinement. Thoroughly socialized flies then needed more sleep than solitary flies, and this sleep resulted in synaptic downscaling. The synapses of flies that were sleep deprived weren't downscaled, supporting the idea that sleep is essential for this process.

Support for the synaptic homeostasis model isn't limited to flies. Cirelli, Tononi, and colleagues have conducted a series of experiments in humans, all of which point in the same direction. For a start, when humans spend hours and hours training on a hand-eye coordination task that is known to involve one specific area of the motor cortex, they subsequently get more sleep slow waves in exactly this cortical area—suggesting that these high-amplitude oscillations are needed for the targeted downscaling of those overpotentiated synapses.[3] Conversely, if people are asked to wear an arm sling that prevents them from using one arm and hand, they subsequently show *less* slow waves in the cortical areas associated with these particular limbs.[4] Finally, the same research group tried to artificially potentiate synapses in a specific bit of the neocortex using a stimulation technique called transcranial magnetic stimulation (in which an electromagnet pulses magnetism at targeted brain areas—through the scalp/ skull, etc.—inducing random cell firing in the target region).[5] This led not only to the desired potentiation of synapses in this region but also to an increase in the number of slow waves which occurred there early in the night—once again supporting the idea that localized potentiation leads to localized slow waves, until the potentiation has been reduced to normal levels.

The targeted slow waves in these experiments typically predict the extent to which performance improves across the night of sleep. This is critical to the idea that downscaling could facilitate memory consolidation because it clearly shows the memories in question are not simply wiped out by this process. Instead they are somehow refined or strengthened—which brings us back to the concept of tuning a radio and sharpening a signal.

Although we normally think of sleep as a whole-brain phenomenon, the fact that slow wave activity can increase locally in those areas of the brain where synapses are most strongly potentiated seems to suggest this is a simplification. Indeed, it turns out that small areas of the brain can exhibit properties of slow wave sleep even when you're wide awake. During wakefulness, neurons fire irregularly, which is why the EEG—electroencephalography—which measures how brain responses vary over time shows fast irregular oscillations (see chapter 1). When you enter slow wave sleep, this pattern is quite different. Instead of irregular (but fairly constant) firing, neurons have "off" periods when they don't fire and "on" periods when they do, and this combination creates slow waves. Very recent neural recordings in rats have shown that localized areas of the neocortex can exhibit this off/on pattern when a rat is tired (e.g., after it has been awake for a long time), even if the rat is wide awake and active. It looks like small areas of the cortex are slyly napping on the job, without waiting for the whole brain to fall asleep. This impression is emphasized by the fact that the rats do worse at various tasks (in this case reaching out to collect little sugar pills) when parts of the brain are napping in this way.[6]

SUMMING UP

This chapter should have convinced you that, like every good cellar or attic, the brain needs a regular clear-out. The evidence from both flies and humans strongly suggests that this type of synaptic downscaling (or synaptic homeostasis) is part of the function of slow wave sleep. The idea that such cleaning sharpens the signal-to-noise ratio of important memories so they pop out from the background of unwanted garbage provides an initial hypothesis about how sleep may act to facilitate subsequent remembering. In the next two chapters, you'll read about how memories are replayed during sleep and how such replay could relate to dream imagery. We will revisit the idea of synaptic homeostasis and the "memory tuning" hypothesis at the end of chapter 6, where we'll think about how it fits in (or doesn't) with other theories of sleep and memory.

six

how and why memories are "replayed" in sleep

IN THE NEAR FUTURE, YOU MAY AT-
tend a party where you meet a lot of new people and need to
remember all their names. How will you keep them all in mind?
What's the best strategy? One obvious idea would be to repeat
the names to yourself during introductions, saying them out
loud as often as possible as you interact with people at the party.
Rehearsal seems to strengthen memories—and rightly so. The
more often you can associate a face and a name, the more tightly
they become bound together. The problem is that rehearsal also
takes up attention and cognitive resources. It is tricky to rehearse
names while you're carrying on a conversation, conducting business, or flirting with someone attractive. We are normally so busy
performing these (and other) tasks that it would be impossible

for us to find enough time to actively rehearse all of the new information we learn.

What if we could rehearse it all while we sleep? The precious hours of slumber are the one time when our brains aren't busily completing tasks or at least thinking about something specific. This makes sleep the ideal time for rehearsal—and it turns out that we make good use of that time. A recent study of sleepwalking patients illustrated this by showing that sleepwalkers, who are much freer in their movements during sleep than other people, often reenact things they did right before sleep, providing direct evidence for the off-line replay of newly acquired information.[1] Of course this physical reenactment results from a mild sleep disorder. Healthy sleepers don't reenact their memories in this way (just imagine how much energy we would waste if we had to physically act out everything that happened every day during our subsequent sleep). Instead, memory rehearsal during sleep normally occurs at a strictly neural level, so studies have to take a more subtle approach and look at brain activity in order to detect it. To understand these methods, you will need to know a bit more about the structure and function of the brain. I'm therefore going to subject you to a crash course in neuroanatomy and how we measure brain activity.

BASIC BRAIN ANATOMY

In chapter 3 we looked at the brain as a glob of pink-gray jelly, which, when sliced in various directions, turned out to contain different types of material—gray matter, white matter, and even quite distinct patterns of cellular architecture in different regions. In fact, the brain can be divided into hundreds of different structures, each having its own function as well as its own unique cellular architecture and connectivity.

One easy way to think of the brain is in an evolutionary sense, as a highly organized globular mass of neurons that has grown out from the stalk it sits on over many millennia of evolution. The parts of the brain that evolved first are those nearest the stalk, while the newest bits, and thus those that are unique to mammals or even humans, are located toward the outside of the glob, as far as possible from the stalk. As a rule of thumb, the oldest parts control the most fundamental processes, such as regulation of heart rate and body temperature, and are therefore absolutely essential for survival, while the newest parts perform less critical functions, such as those associated with conscious thought (this may not sound optional, but lots of animals survive without it—just think about insects and crustaceans).

The stalk on which the brain sits is of course the spinal cord, which broadens at the top to form the brainstem (Fig. 13). The brainstem controls a host of basic bodily functions such as homeostasis, respiration, swallowing, bladder function, equilibrium, eye movement, facial expressions, posture, and aspects of sleep. Just above the brainstem is the midbrain, which is critical for many metabolic processes and for the control of body temperature, hunger, thirst, fatigue, circadian rhythms, and (again) aspects of sleep. On top of the midbrain sit two symmetrical and quite independent brain hemispheres connected only by a thick fiber tract called the corpus callosum.

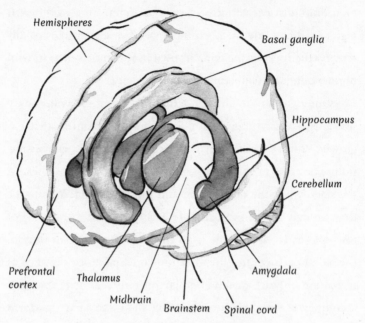

Fig. 13   Gross anatomy of the brain

Within each of these hemispheres, directly on top of the midbrain, sits the thalamus, a roughly spherical structure which receives inputs from most of the brain regions involved in thought, action, and sensation, and which also projects back out to these areas. Because of its ubiquitous connections, the thalamus is often thought of as a "relay station" for the brain. It may act like a sort of telephone operator, allowing different regions to communicate through it when direct connections are not present. Curling around each spherical thalamus is a set of nuclei known as the basal ganglia. These are critically involved in the control of movement, as well as some forms of skill learning. Projecting sideways from the basal ganglia is the hippocampus, which has developed greatly in mammals but is present to some extent in all vertebrates. The hippocampus is critical for many types of memory and is especially involved in navigation. Finally, projecting forward and down from the basal ganglia is the olfactory bulb, which receives direct input from the nose and sends this on to the rest of the brain.

All of the brain structures mentioned so far are part of the evolutionarily "old" brain shared by all vertebrates. Although these regions may have changed in size, shape, and importance across the millennia, they are present in some form in every creature with a backbone. The mammalian brain is typically larger, with respect to body size, than that of other vertebrates. The brain of any given mammal will be roughly twice as large as that of a bird and ten times as large as that of a reptile with the same body size. The main reason for this size difference is the dramatic enlargement and structural alteration of the front part of the brain, called the forebrain. The mammalian forebrain is characterized by a complex six-layered structure called the neocortex, which is not present in other vertebrates.

In humans, the neocortex is densely folded to provide extra surface area. Although part of the forebrain, the neocortex coats the entire outside of our globular mass, including front, back, and any areas underneath where there is space in the skull. This part of the brain is literally packed into every remaining nook and cranny. The neocortex is the seat of higher thought—executive control, attention, and the ability to reason. It is likely that it also contains the key to consciousness, but this remains to be established. Along the edges of the neocortex, several structures that were present before the expansion of this huge organ swamped the rest of the brain have also developed and taken on new forms. These include the hippocampus and amygdala.

For our purposes, it is important to understand the neocortex in more detail. First, there are principle areas for touch, vision, hearing, smell, and taste. These are literally separate geographic regions. The visual cortex is in the lower back part of the brain, the auditory cortex is in the middle of the sides, and the tactile cortex starts right in the middle of the top and runs down the sides from there (Fig. 14). Each of these areas responds uniquely to a particular input—so if we show the animal a light, we'll find activity in the visual cortex, playing music will lead to activity in the auditory cortex, and stroking the animal (or prodding it) will activate the tactile (also known as somatosensory) cortex. Just in front of the somatosensory cortex is a region that

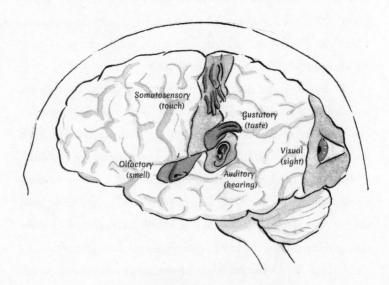

Fig. 14 Sensory cortices of the brain

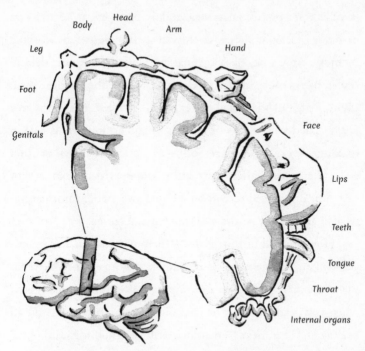

Fig. 15   *The somatosensory homunculus (above) is located within a cross-section of the neocortex (rectangular grey box below).*

specializes in motor control. The neurons here are directly connected to bodily muscles using just one synapse, so they have very immediate control over our movements. Both the motor and somatosensory cortices are arranged as a map of the body—each of these is called a homunculus, which means "little man." The name is apt because, if drawn out (Fig. 15), the body map that exists in each of these regions would look like a little man (or woman, depending of course upon whose brain we are talking about).

In front of the somatosensory and motor cortices is a largish area that extends across the whole front of the brain. This is called the prefrontal cortex and is believed to be the seat of higher thought processes as well as functions like working memory, reasoning, decision making, and self-control. Behind the somatosensory cortex, and extending all the way down to the top edge of the visual cortex, is the parietal lobe. This area is associated with attention but also plays an important role in making associations between other cortical areas as well as other tasks like mathematical calculation and spatial awareness. For instance, if we need to combine visual and tactile information, we will almost always draw on the parietal cortex.

How does all of this relate to memory? The answer is simple—when you remember a situation, the parts of the brain that were activated by sensory inputs (taste, touch, smell, etc.) when you originally experienced the situation become active all over again. This means a memory with both auditory and visual components, such as talking to a friend, will elicit essentially the same neural responses in the auditory and visual cortices as happened when you had that conversation in the first place. Your brain is literally reliving the memory. This is critical for the concept of memory consolidation, and it is also critical for the idea of memory replay during sleep, as you'll soon see. First, however, let me explain some of the techniques we scientists use to examine brain responses.

MEASURING BRAIN ACTIVITY

What does it mean when we say a piece of the brain is active? This quite literally means the neurons in that particular area are firing more action potentials than they normally would. In some brain areas, action potentials are more or less chronic, so saying the region has become active is relative: It really means the frequency or density of action potentials is increased.

How do we know about these action potentials? There are lots of ways. The most fine-grained method involves sticking an electrode, which is essentially a very tiny and sensitive metal spike that easily picks up electrical signals, into the brain (and in some cases even directly into the cell) and measuring changes in electrical potential. Although recordings with sharp electrodes of this type allow a detailed understanding of how the cells in a particular area act in terms of electrical responses, it is not so helpful if you want to examine the overall activity of hundreds or thousands of cells, some of which might be nowhere near the tip of your little probe. Perhaps more importantly, it isn't always practical to put electrodes into all of the brains we'd want to study. You probably wouldn't feel too kindly toward an eager neuroscientist who wanted to drill a hole in your skull, screw a metal cannula to it, and spend hours poking around in your brain with these little spears—doing irreparable damage while she was at it. Oddly enough, this lack of enthusiasm is shared by many people, including the university students upon whom many neuroscience experiments are carried out.

Instead of using these needlelike intracranial (or intracellular) electrodes, neuroscientists can also use flat electrodes, which resemble a small coin with a wire attached, glued to the scalp. These pick up changes in electrical field in an analogous manner to the pointy intracranial variety, but they are completely noninvasive and can be taken off in a few moments, leaving only a sticky legacy of electroconductive paste—which means participants often have to wash their hair, but there is no lasting damage. The use of electrodes on the scalp to measure fluctuating electrical fields in the brain is called electroencephalography, or EEG. EEG is a fantastic way of capturing the quick-changing activity of the brain in real time and is particularly convenient for measuring sleep, as we saw in chapter 1. The main downside to EEG is its profound lack of spatial precision. Electrical potentials measured on the scalp may have percolated from almost anywhere in the brain. Dense arrays of 256 or more electrodes, spaced close together all over the head, are sometimes used to try and increase precision, but even with this high-density recording, it is still difficult to be certain where the electrical activity is coming from.

In order to get a better idea about the location of neural responses, scientists have to use different techniques, and one of the most common is functional magnetic resonance imaging, or fMRI, which exploits the electrical properties of oxygenated blood to measure the changes in blood flow which typically accompany strong neural activity. Like EEG, fMRI is totally noninvasive. Unlike EEG, however, it is extremely spatially precise and can show us where changes in blood flow are occurring within a couple of millimeters. The big catch with fMRI, however, is that it is slow. Although the spatial resolution is good, the temporal resolution is terrible since it can take anywhere between 3 and 12 seconds for blood flow to increase after a region of the brain initially becomes active. Another snag is that fMRI only picks up relatively huge changes in activity, since these are the ones that trigger an influx of oxygenated blood. While the sharp, pointy electrodes our neuroscientist wanted to stick deep into your brain would have been sensitive to activity in one or two cells right by the electrode tip, fMRI tells us about the mass activation of thousands of neurons.

All of these techniques can be used to help us understand how memory lodges itself in our brains and with what modifications. So far, as described above, we have one technique that can only measure a few cells at a time (and has the downside of causing permanent brain damage); another that tells us when the brain responds but can't really tell us where; and a third that tells us where, but not when, neural activity is happening. It doesn't sound like such a promising arsenal, does it? Well, it really isn't that promising. Neuroscientists are trying to reverse-engineer the most complicated computer ever designed using these tools in different combinations (plus a few more I haven't mentioned), and it really isn't easy, but the potential reward, or perhaps the fascinating nature of the problem, keeps them pushing forward.

SPONTANEOUS MEMORY
REPLAY DURING SLEEP

We have said that the neocortex contains areas that respond specifically to things like vision, sound, touch, and so forth. It isn't much of a jump to realize that some combination of these areas is active pretty much all the time, and the exact pattern of activity depends on what you are experiencing. So, if you are running on the beach with sand under your feet, sun on your skin, the sound of waves in your ears, sky in your eyes, and the smell of salt in your nostrils, then all of the appropriate areas of the brain (touch sensation, audition, vision, olfaction, etc.) will be activated to allow you to experience these sensations. This activity, plus responses in a few regions of the brain used to pull things together, makes up your experience of that particular moment in time. A slightly bigger jump is needed to realize this pattern of sensory activity isn't just the basis of experiences when you have them. It is also the basis of your memories.

One prominent theory suggests the experiences which are coded into various sensory areas of the neocortex need to be linked together to form complete representations of the episode, and this linking is initially performed by the hippocampus. When we remember these episodes in the absence of sensory inputs (for instance, when lying in bed with the lights off and silence all around), the hippocampus triggers activity in all of the appropriate sensory areas needed to allow you to relive the original experience. It has "remembered" the association between these specific sensations and linked them together. Once triggered, these sensory areas activate in much the same way as they would if you were exposed to the original stimuli all over again. Your brain is replaying the memory just as you might replay a video or piece of music (Fig. 16).

The analogy with music is actually quite useful, especially if you think of the cortex as a piano keyboard with different keys representing different sensory inputs. The keys are all there to be played all the time, but they only have a noticeable impact when they are pressed, and only a few are pressed at any given time. If we think of the memory of running on the beach as a beautiful piece of music, a standard view of memory would suggest the score for this music is initially stored in the hippocampus. When the memory is relived, the hippocampus sends triggers to

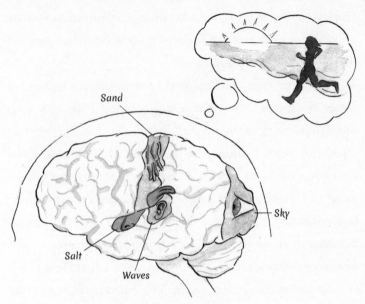

Fig. 16   Memory replay in the sensory cortices

all of the relevant piano keys (areas of neocortex) in the correct order and with the correct timing to produce the music. So, for example, the different aspects of running on the beach, such as the feeling of sand on your feet, the color of the ocean, and the smell of salty air, are stored in different cortical regions. The hippocampus is in charge of triggering all of these elements to allow you to re-experience the memory, and the neocortex merely provides the various notes on demand.

At the beginning of the chapter, I said the brain replays memories while you are asleep. Does this mean your hippocampus and neocortex could actually be performing a concert while you snooze? The answer is yes. Furthermore, while some such replay might manifest itself as a dream, there is fairly strong evidence that much of it is subconscious. This means you are probably not even aware of the symphony which is being played in your brain as you slumber.

The more often a set of neural representations is used together as a group the more tightly they become bound to each other (think back to the rhyme "neurons that fire together wire together," which I introduced in chapter 3). This means that even when you aren't aware of it, repeatedly rehearsing a specific pattern of neural activity is bound to influence the associations between different brain regions. The replaying of memories during sleep therefore provides one possible key to the mystery of how sleep promotes consolidation. Let's take a closer look.

The most convincing evidence for memory replay during sleep comes from a very special population of cells, called place cells, which respond when an animal (human, rat, or other) is in a specific location, and only when it is in that location. As you move around a room or other open space, different place cells will fire. However, each time you go back to a previous location, the cell that fired last time you were there fires again. So these cells are associated with a particular place, and once they've become associated, they don't switch. Why is this useful for studying memory replay?

Here's why: When you move along a route in space, a specific set of place cells will fire in the same order: cell 1 for the start, cell 2 for the next location, cell 3 for the next, and so on until you get to the finishing point (say, cell 4). The next time you move along that route, the same cells will fire in the same order—and the next time, and the next, and so forth (Fig. 17, top). Moving along that route is associated with a highly stereotypical and easily identifiable sequence of place cell firing. If you are a rat learning to run through a maze, and you later replay that experience in your sleep, what will happen? Exactly the same sequence of cells that fired when you took the correct route through the maze will fire again in exactly the same order when you rehearse this information (Fig. 17, bottom). Because

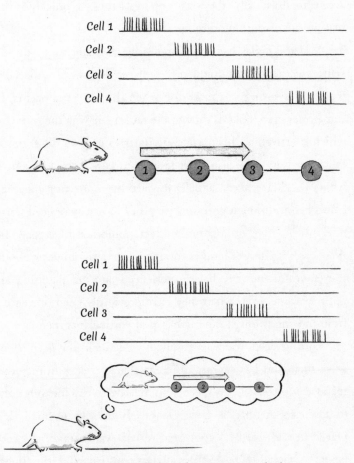

Fig. 17   Place cells firing during movement (top);
memory replay in place cells (bottom)

this sequential firing is so distinct, it provides the perfect tool for examining neural replay during sleep. In fact, studies in which electrodes were implanted in the hippocampus have shown that rats who are highly trained on running through a maze or track replay the sequence of cells associated with running through that environment spontaneously, both while they are awake but resting and while they are asleep. When they are awake these replays accelerate drastically (they occur up to 21 times as quickly as the real-life act of running through the maze).

Wakeful replay has other interesting characteristics—for instance, sequences are frequently replayed backward, especially if the rat is sitting at a food dish when this rehearsal occurs. It sometimes even looks as though the rat is reviewing the route by which it arrived at this particularly tasty (and rewarding) point in space. Rats have also been known to construct new routes which they have never actually traveled by connecting together a number of different corridors that they have experienced separately into a new, usually more direct, combined trajectory.[2] In these cases it almost seems as though the rats are thinking about the environment they have experienced and are planning an optimal route, even when they have previously been prevented from moving through the maze in that particular way.

During sleep, route replay mainly occurs in the deep, slow wave stage and has slightly different characteristics from route replay during wake. It is speeded up relative to real life, but only to about seven times as fast as reality. Routes are normally replayed in a forward (as compared to backward) trajectory, and (so far as we know) new routes are not constructed during these replays. Fascinatingly, the number of replays predicts the extent to which rats improve on these maze tasks across sleep, providing strong support for the idea that these replays are associated with neuroplasticity and consolidation during sleep. Disrupting replay by injecting tiny amounts of electrical current into the relevant region of hippocampus just when a replay is likely to occur prevents consolidation since it abolishes the usual overnight improvement on memory tasks, which further supports the importance of these events for consolidation.[3]

Although place cells provide an excellent and easily verifiable marker of replay, they are not the only cells that show this pattern. Recordings in the visual and somatosensory cortices, as well as other areas such as the basal ganglia, are also consistent with the replay of sensory inputs experienced in wake, although it seems likely these responses are triggered by replay in the hippocampus (e.g., in the manner of our piano concerto). There has been only one report of replay during REM sleep, but this suggested a much more extensive and complete concerto, lasting longer and containing many elements of the experience, e.g., triggering activity in areas associated with arousal levels as well as sensory inputs. Could such extensive replay during REM sleep actually be a dream, just captured in electrodes? This has been suggested, but we will never know the answer—the rats involved in that experiment are all long since dead, and none of them was in the habit of reporting their dreams anyway.

We humans also show memory replay during sleep, but we haven't been studied as much as rats since, as mentioned earlier, we tend not to like having people poke around in our brains with electrodes. Work with fMRI shows that the parts of the human hippocampus which are active when we explore a maze in a video game are also active during our slow wave sleep the following night. The extent of this activity predicts how much our ability to navigate around the maze is improved the next day. More excitingly, there is at least a bit of evidence that we can trigger replay by presenting cues during sleep that are linked to the memory we want to consolidate. This has worked with smells and sounds, both of which seem to trigger consolidation since the memories they pertain to were remembered better after they were presented during sleep; see chapter 12 for more on this.

MEMORY REPLAY AND CONSOLIDATION

Thinking back to that infamous party at which you are going to have to remember so many new names, the above discussion seems to suggest that you are not only likely to rehearse those names while you're at the party, you're also likely to rehearse them during your subsequent sleep. This rehearsal will involve reactivation of the brain regions that were associated with learning the name/face pairing—so that means parts of your temporal lobe (associated with words) and your visual cortex (associated with faces) will be concurrently active. The process of repeatedly activating neurons in both of these areas will cause them to become more tightly bound. Although the name and face areas may initially have been linked together via the hippocampus, enough reactivations should eventually ensure that activity in one would lead to activity in the other. If you happen to see one of your new contacts a few times after the party (or just think about her a lot), you will probably remember her name easily each time

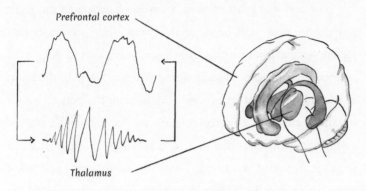

Prefrontal cortex

Thalamus

Fig. 18   The active systems consolidation hypothesis

you see her face—or vice versa. Although you probably won't
monitor these reactivations in your brain, a neuroscientist who
wanted to study the consolidation process would be able to do so
either invasively, by sticking electrodes into your cortex, or less
traumatically by using fMRI and/or EEG to get an idea of what
was going on in there.

Is sleep only good for this type of consolidation because it
provides a time when our brains aren't busy doing other things?
Some scientists think there's nothing too special about sleep, except that no new information is coming in, which means existing memories can more easily be processed. Others, however,
take an entirely different view and think that memories are actively processed by sleep in a way that isn't possible during wake.
Memory replay is critical for these ideas, but of course memory
replay also occurs during wake (e.g., you could make a conscious
decision to rehearse the names and faces of everyone you met at
the party). What does sleep add that wake can't?

The active systems consolidation model suggests the high-amplitude, slow oscillations of slow wave sleep serve a critical function for memory replay.[4] You'll remember that in chapter 1 I likened these large amplitude, slow-frequency waves to the huge, rhythmic stirrings of a Loch Ness Monster in the bottom of our hypothetical lake. When picked up by flat electrodes on the scalp, huge responses like this are a sure sign that many, many neurons are acting in unison. These big oscillations in electrical signal mean that hosts of brain cells are first moving toward the electrical state in which they will fire an action potential (the difference between electrical charges inside and outside the cell is getting smaller) and then moving away from that electrical state (the difference between electrical charge inside and outside the cell is getting bigger, meaning the cell is unlikely to fire). You'll remember from chapter 3 that these changes are achieved by moving electrically charged particles into or out of the cell. The point is that these slow waves influence the moments at which cells in the brain can fire. By pushing the cells first *toward* the state in which they can fire and then *away from* that state, slow waves make sure that if cells are going to fire they all do it at roughly the same time. Cortical cells in the areas associated with the memory obviously have to fire when memories are replayed (exactly as discussed earlier in this chapter). What these slow waves do with respect to memory is control the timing of when this happens. Specifically, these slow waves coordinate replays so they take place at more or less the same time wherever they are happening in the brain. This is thought to be particularly important if replays involve structures that are anatomically far apart, such as the hippocampus and neocortical processing areas, which you might use for remembering the link between a face and a voice. The slow waves percolate throughout all of these regions, providing a basic STOP or GO signal that makes sure all of the replay occurs at the same time. Remembering the rhyme, "neurons which fire together wire together," it is easy to see why the temporal synchronization of replays is essential if this activity is going to eventually strengthen memory representations by strengthening the synaptic connections between neurons involved in representing a specific face and neurons involved in representing a specific voice. The temporal coordination of replays may also ensure that information gets passed efficiently from one structure to another (e.g., from the hippocampus to the neocortex), and that the cells in the neocortex are in a state in which replay will have a maximal effect in terms of strengthening connections between neurons (Madonna's face and voice) and thus strengthening memory representations (if Madonna phones you up, you'll know who it is).

My sharp-eyed readers may have picked up a contradiction here. In chapter 5 I explained the idea of synaptic homeostasis—that is, downscaling or weakening of synaptic strengths that happens across the board during slow wave sleep.[5] I also explained that this downscaling is thought to strengthen memories by removing background noise, so the strongest (and hopefully most important) part of the signal is maintained while weaker junk signal is lost. I drew an analogy between this process and turning down the volume on a staticky radio. The idea that synapses are actually strengthened during slow wave sleep as a result of memory replay is a direct contradiction of this synaptic downscaling principle. This has caused a lot of problems for the study of sleep and memory, especially as a huge number of studies have shown that synapses *are* downscaled and not strengthened during slow wave sleep. However, recent work has provided evidence that a small proportion of synapses can also be strengthening during slow wave sleep, so it seems likely that both processes could be happening at the same time. Slow wave sleep does lead to a global downscaling of synapses and with it to a reduction in the neural noise that makes it hard to separate real memories from garbage. However, it also coordinates the replay of memories and could well be associated with the type of targeted strengthening proposed here. So this sleep stage essentially has a double-whammy effect on memory, both removing background noise and strengthening target information. No wonder you remember things better after they've been replayed during slow wave sleep!

SUMMING UP

This chapter has explained how memories are replayed during sleep and why that is important for memory. To really understand memory replay, it is important to realize that different parts of the brain represent different types of sensation (like vision, hearing, and touch). It is also important to have a feel for the ways in which we can measure brain activity—with sharp electrodes inserted into the brain, with flat coin-like electrodes on the scalp for EEG, or with fMRI. After going over these basics, we also went through some of the strongest evidence that neural replay does actually occur during sleep. This comes from both location-specific place cells in rats and obvious performance improvements after sleep in humans. Finally, we saw why neural replay is important for memory consolidation, and why the huge electrical oscillations of slow wave sleep are thought to facilitate this process by making certain everything happens at just the right time. The next chapter is about dreaming and provides a completely different angle on the idea of neural replay during sleep.

seven

what is dreaming and what does it tell us about memory?

YOU ARE TERRIFIED AND RUNNING along a dark, narrow corridor. Something very evil and scary is chasing you, but you're not sure why. Your fear is compounded by the fact that your feet won't do what you want—it feels like they are moving through molasses. The pursuer is gaining, but when it finally catches you, the whole scene vanishes . . . and you wake up.

Almost by definition, a dream is something you are aware of at some level. It may be fragmentary, disconnected, and illogical, but if you aren't aware of it during sleep then it isn't a dream. Many people will protest, "I never remember my dreams!," but that is a different matter entirely. Failing to remember a dream later on when you're awake doesn't mean you weren't aware of it when it occurred. It just means the experience was never really carved into your memory, has decayed in storage, or isn't accessible for easy call back.

We all intuitively know what a dream is, but you'll be surprised to learn there's no universally accepted definition of dreaming. One fairly safe catch-all is "all perceptions, thoughts, or emotions experienced during sleep."[1] Because this is very broad, there are also several different ways of rating, ranking, and scoring dreams. For example, one uses an eight-point rating system from 0 (no dream) to 7 ("an extremely long sequence of 5 or more stages").[2]

PHYSICAL BASES OF DREAMS

But let me backtrack. One aim of neuroscience is to map the brain loci of thoughts and mental experiences. Everything we see, imagine, or think about is linked to neural responses somewhere in the brain. Dreams also have a home. We saw in chapter 6 that neural activity in the primary sensory areas of the neocortex produces the impression of sensory perception. This means that neurons firing in the primary visual cortex create the illusion of seeing things, neurons firing in the primary auditory area create the illusion of hearing things, and so forth. If that firing occurs at random, these perceptions can feel like crazy, randomly fragmented hallucinations. It is easy to imagine that the random imagery and sensations created in this way could be woven together to create a complex, multisensory hallucination which we might call a dream.

In 1977 two Harvard scientists, Allan Hobson and Bob Mc-Carley, proposed a theory about how dreams occur called the activation-synthesis model.[3] This draws on knowledge of sleep physiology to propose that dreams are generated in precisely the way described above. It turns out that chaotic firing of neurons in the brainstem is a core characteristic of REM sleep. Because these brainstem neurons communicate with the neocortex, their chaotic firing could trigger responses in the primary sensory and motor areas. The activation-synthesis model proposes that the brain may combine and synthesize these neocortical responses to create a story (Fig. 19). This explanation works well at the physiological level: We know the nightmarish dreams epileptic people

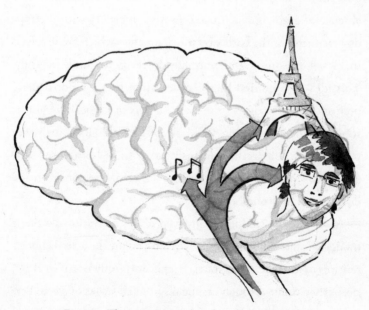

Fig. 19   The activation synthesis hypothesis of dreaming

sometimes have are caused by partial seizures which entail high-intensity, chaotic activity in the brain's emotional system. In fact, electrical stimulation applied externally to the cortex can lead to dreamlike perceptions even during wakefulness.[4] Both the data from epileptic patients and the electrical stimulation data show that chaotically triggered brainstem activity can lead to the subjective perception of a dream.

Allan Hobson extended the activation-synthesis model by taking the pharmacology of sleep into account. He proposed that high levels of the neurotransmitter acetylcholine, in combination with the low levels of aminergic neurotransmitters such as norepinephrine which occur during REM sleep (see chapter 4), could cause a sense of bizarreness (e.g., unusual juxtapositions, distortions, illogical reasoning, and sudden scene changes). The absence of aminergic neurotransmitters interferes with the top-down control of the cortex by the brain areas which are involved in higher reasoning and normally force us to think logically. This idea is supported by the observation that the dorsolateral prefrontal cortex, one of the main centers of higher thought, is relatively inactive during REM sleep. In fact, Hobson drew a parallel between dreams and psychoses, since both entail hallucinations and illusions, as well as abnormal responses in the dorsolateral prefrontal cortex.

Unfortunately, Hobson and McCarley's activation-synthesis model is less convincing when we think about the actual characteristics of dreams. For a start, dreams don't only occur in REM sleep; they occur throughout the night in all stages of sleep. Perhaps more telling is the content of dreams. Studies have shown that many dreams are sensible, logical, and thematic, though potentially somewhat disconnected. Could chaotic neural activity really produce this pattern? And what about those recurrent nightmares that haunt us night after night? How could these be caused by semi-random brainstem responses? These combined characteristics of dreams (occurrence throughout the night, recurrence, and in some cases thematic logic) imply that they are generated in a structured way.

Not only are dreams not generated by chaotic brain activity, there is also strong evidence against the idea that primary sensory areas orchestrate dreams. Scientists often learn about how the body and the mind work by studying patients who are damaged or deficient in some way. When people suffer damage to the primary visual or sensory cortices, this causes no apparent deficit to vision or touch in dreams, even though it may cause either complete or partial blindness and inability to feel the things they actually do touch. A good example of this comes from people who have massive lesions to their primary sensory and motor cortices which can lead to paralysis of the arm, leg, and trunk on one side of the body (this is called hemiplegia). Amazingly enough, people with hemiplegia still enjoy normal dream imagery about bilateral movement in all of these body parts. Similarly, aphasic patients, who have great trouble talking due to extensive damage to the areas of the brain that control speech, have completely normal speech-related dreams. The experiences of these brain-damaged patients show us that the primary sensory and motor cortices are not responsible for generating imagery in dreams. Instead, dream imagery appears to be created in a more cognitively mediated fashion which involves the higher-level sensory and motor association cortices, which process sensory signals in a more refined way. For example, damage to the visual association cortex (which processes more complex visual information such as movement, orientation, color, size, and shape, and which normally only engages when you are paying attention to what your eyes are seeing) can lead to a complete loss of visual imagery in dreams.

With the great advantage of hindsight, some modern critics of the activation-synthesis model have suggested that, in its enthusiasm for the role of random activity in the brainstem in triggering the neocortical activity which underpins dreams, this model may have overinterpreted the reduced activity in the dorsolateral prefrontal cortex during REM sleep and not paid enough attention to other areas of the prefrontal cortex which are highly activated in REM sleep. Examples of such areas are the anterior cingulate, which is known to play an important control function in the brain (for instance, keeping the wayward amygdala in check in frightening situations); and the ventromedial prefrontal cortex, which is thought to be responsible for the sense of self. With these structures online in REM, it seems odd to assume that the dreams which occur during this sleep stage are generated in an entirely uncontrolled fashion.

A newer model of dreams was proposed by Mark Solms, then at the Royal London School of Medicine, in 2000. This model argues against Hobson and McCarley's activation-synthesis ideas by suggesting that, far from being caused by chaotic activity in the brainstem and cortex, dreams are actually generated by the thinking part of the brain. Solms reviewed data from brain-damaged patients and discovered that people with lesions to the ventromedial prefrontal cortex seem to lose their ability to dream. His work suggests that the brain's reward system, which originates in the midbrain and connects through the ventromedial prefrontal cortex as it projects upward to the rest of the brain, provides the basis for dreams. Lesions to the ventromedial prefrontal region dramatically disrupt this system. Chemical stimulation of the reward system (for instance, through the administration of L-dopa, a drug which can be converted to dopamine, the brain's primary neurotransmitter of reward) causes both psychotic symptoms and excessive, un-usually vivid dreaming. Blocking the action of dopamine using drugs—such as haloperidol, which clogs up receptors for this neurotransmitter—inhibits excessively vivid dreaming. Inciden-tally, haloperidol is often used to treat schizophrenia precisely because of its ability to inhibit psychoses.

Interestingly, the ventromedial prefrontal cortex, which Solms found to be so important for dreaming, is the same part of the prefrontal cortex that was often intentionally destroyed in order to restore the sanity of the patient in the heyday of invasive psychiatric procedures. It turns out that 70 to 90 percent of such prefrontal lobotomies also resulted in a complete loss of dream-ing, which once more supports the parallel between dreaming and psychosis, as well as the importance of the reward system for dreaming.

In addition to the ventromedial prefrontal cortex, Solms found that lesions to the three-way junction between tempo-ral cortex (which mediates sound processing and also general knowledge), parietal cortex (which mediates attention), and occipital cortex (which mediates vision) also abolished dreams. This region is important for mental imagery, so it isn't surprising that lesions here disrupt dreaming.

DREAMS ARE LIMITED BY
COGNITIVE ABILITY AND STATE

Even among the healthy, not everyone is capable of normal dreams. The complexity, length, and thematic coherence of dreams all seem to be partially determined by the general cognitive capacity of the dreamer. For instance, there is evidence that autistic people have shorter dreams with fewer elements in them, and they recall less detail about the dreams they do have. This suggests a possible link between the ability to dream and a person's general capacity for creative, imaginative, emotional thinking. In a similar vein, children younger than five years old tend to have unstructured dreams with poor narrative development; in the dreams of five- to eight-year-olds, these properties are predicted by measures of visuospatial intelligence.[5] Interestingly, people with schizophrenia have brief dreams with limited hallucinatory content. These dreams contain a lot of aggression, and this is usually directed toward the dreamer. Particularly violent dreams can precede a psychotic scene in wake, and patients with very severe symptoms can have trouble distinguishing between wake and dreaming.[6] The dreams of people with depression vary a lot. Some studies have shown that depressed people have short, bland dreams. Other observations have suggested that they have more negative and masochistic dreams. These differences are probably due to the fact that depression is a hugely diverse condition, and different studies probably included people with different subtypes of depression.

DO DREAMS SERVE A PURPOSE?

In contrast to the activation-synthesis model, which views dreams as epiphenomena—a simple by-product of neural processes in sleep—other scientists have suggested that dreams serve an important function. As usual in psychology, there are lots of different ideas about what this function could be. Sigmund Freud's suggestion that dreams express forbidden desires is of course the most famous of these, but there are lots of other theories about what dreams might do, many with more empirical support than the Freudian view. For example, the threat simulation hypothesis suggests that dreams may provide a sort of virtual reality simulation in which we can rehearse threatening situations, even if we don't remember the dreams. Presumably, this rehearsal would lead to better real-life responses, so the rehearsal is adaptive.[7] Evidence supporting this comes from the large proportion of dreams which include a threatening situation (more than 70 percent in some studies) and the fact that this percentage is much higher than the incidence of threats in the dreamer's actual daytime life. Furthermore, studies of children in two different areas of Palestine show that those who live in a more threatening environment also have a much higher incidence of threat in their dreams. Reactions to these threats are almost always relevant and sensible, so the rehearsal (if that's what it is) clearly involves plausible solutions, again suggesting that they provide a kind of valid simulation of potential real-life scenarios.

Another suggestion is that dreams influence the way you feel the next day, either in terms of mood or more basic bodily states. Forcing people to remember the nastier dreams from their REM sleep definitely puts them in a foul mood, and nightmares (defined as very negative dreams which can wake you up) may even lead to ongoing mood problems. On the other hand, there is also evidence that dreams could help to regulate long-term mood. For instance, a study of dreams in divorced women showed that those who dreamed about their ex-husbands more often were better adapted to the divorce.[8] Amazingly enough, dreams also seem able to influence physiological state: One study showed that people who were deprived of water before they slept, but then drank in their dreams, felt less thirsty when they woke up.[9]

The content of dreams can be influenced in lots of different ways. For instance, recent work has shown that sleepers tend to initiate pleasant dreams if nice smells are wafted at them in REM sleep, and they have negative or unhappy dreams if stinky, unpleasant smells are sent their way.[10] Some people can achieve lucid dreaming, in which they control the sequence of events in their dream, and evidence suggests that these techniques can be learned by intensive practice and training. All of this is highly tantalizing, of course, because (though it tells us nothing at all about the original evolved purpose of dreams) it suggests we might not only be able to set ourselves up for pleasant experiences while we sleep, but we might also eventually be able to use these techniques to treat mood disorders, phobias, and other psychological problems. We already know that hypnotic suggestion can cause people to incorporate snakes, spiders, or other things about which they have phobias into their dreams, and—when

combined with more benign forms of these menacing objects—
such incorporation helps to remove the phobia. Hypnotic suggestion can also make dreams more pleasant, and mental imagery
practiced during the day can be used to modify (and often nul-
lify) persistent nightmares.

There is little evidence that people actually learn during
their dreams. The fact that they can learn during sleep is a different matter, but dreams themselves don't appear to be a good
forum for imprinting new information into the hippocampus
(after all, we don't even remember our dreams most of the time).
Studies of language learning illustrate this well. Although learning efficiency is predicted by an increase in the percentage of the
night that is spent in REM, the dreams which are experienced
during this extra REM don't have much to do with language. If
they relate to it at all they are most often about the frustration
of not being able to understand something and not about the
mechanics of how to construct or decode a sentence.

MEMORIES IN DREAMS

What's the most recent dream you can remember? Was anyone
you know in it? Did it happen in a place you know well? Were you
doing something familiar? Most dreams incorporate fragments of
experiences from our waking lives. It's common to dream about
disconnected snippets like a particular person, place, or activity.
But do dreams ever replay complete memories—for instance,
the last time you saw your mother, including the place, activities, and people? Memories like this are called episodic because
they represent whole episodes instead of just fragments; studies

of dreaming show that these types of memories *are* sometimes replayed in sleep, but it is quite rare (around 2 percent of dreams contain such memories, according to one study).[11] Most of our dreams just recombine fragments of waking life. These fragments are relatively familiar and reflect the interests and concerns of the dreamer. This means cyclists dream about cycling, teachers dream about teaching, and bankers dream about money.

Some researchers have capitalized upon dream reports to gain insight into the process by which memories are immediately incorporated (i.e., in the first night after they were initially experienced). Freud famously referred to this as "day-residues." One study showed day residues appear in 65 to 70 percent of single dream reports.[12] On the other hand, a more recently described phenomenon called the dream-lag effect refers to the extraordinary observation that, after its initial appearance as a day residue, the likelihood that a specific memory will be incorporated into dreams decreases steadily across the next few nights after the memory was formed, then increases again across the following few nights (Fig. 20).

Thus, it is very common for memories to be incorporated into dreams on the first night after they were initially experienced (if I have a car crash today, I'm likely to dream about it tonight). The likelihood of such incorporation decreases gradually across the next few nights, with few memories incorporated into dreams three to five days after they occurred. Extraordinarily, however, the probability that a memory will be incorporated into a dream increases again on nights six and seven after it was initially experienced. What is going on here? Why are memories less likely to be incorporated into dreams three to five days after

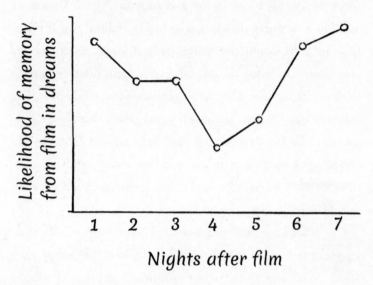

Fig. 20   The dream-lag effect in memory for a film

they originally occurred than six to seven days afterward? One possibility relates to the need for consolidation. Memories may be inaccessible at this stage because they are being processed in some way which takes them temporarily "offline." Notably, this effect is only true for people who report vivid dreams, and it also appears to only be true of REM dreams. As with most research, the dream-lag effect raises more questions than it answers.

WHY DO WE HAVE DIFFERENT KINDS OF DREAMS AT DIFFERENT STAGES OF THE NIGHT?

Dreams aren't all the same. Everyone is aware of the difference between good and bad dreams, but we don't tend to notice that some dreams are more logical and structured while others are more bizarre. Some dreams are so highly realistic that it is difficult to convince ourselves they aren't real, while others are fuzzy and indistinct. Some dreams are fragmented, jumping rapidly from one topic to another, while others move forward in a more coherent story. Recent analyses have suggested that these differences are far from random; instead they may be driven by the physiology of various brain states and the extent to which structures like the hippocampus and neocortex are in communication during different sleep stages.

Dreams occur in all stages of sleep, but they seem to become increasingly fragmented as the night progresses. In general, they appear to be constructed out of a mishmash of prior experience. As mentioned above, dreams contain disconnected memory fragments: places we've been, faces we've seen, situations that are partly familiar. These fragments can either be pasted together in a semi-random mess or organized in a structured and realistic way. The dreams that occur in non-REM sleep tend to be shorter but more cohesive than REM dreams, and often they relate to things that just happened the day before. REM dreams that occur early in the night often also reflect recent waking experiences, but they are more fragmented than their non-REM counterparts. Conversely, REM dreams that occur late in the night are typically much more bizarre and disjointed.

Simply thinking about where these memory fragments are coming from and how they are connected together may provide an explanation for the difference between early and late-night dreams. The various elements of an episode are thought to be stored in the neocortex, but they are not necessarily linked together to form a complete representation. For example, if your memory of having dinner last night involves memories about a specific place, specific sounds, specific actions, and maybe even memories about other people who were there, each of these bits of information is represented by a different area of the neocortex. Even though they combine together to make up a complete memory, these various neocortical areas may not be directly interlinked. Instead, the hippocampus keeps track of such connections and forms the appropriate linkages, at least while the memory is relatively fresh. However, communication between the neocortex and hippocampus is disrupted during sleep, so this process is also disrupted. During REM sleep, both the hippocampus and those parts of the neocortex which are involved in a current dream are strongly active—but they don't appear to be in communication. Instead, responses in the neocortex occur independently, without hippocampal input, so they must relate to memory fragments rather than linked multisensory representations. Essentially, when memories which have been stored in the neocortex are accessed or activated during REM, they remain fragmentary instead of drawing in other aspects of the same memory to form a complete episodic replay. These fragments aren't linked together in the way they might be if you thought of the same place while you were awake (or indeed in non-REM sleep). For instance, cortical representations of both someone who was present for your dinner last night and of the place where it was held may be triggered, but these will not necessarily be linked together, and they may not be linked to the idea of dinner or eating at all. Instead, seemingly unrelated characters and events may be activated in conjunction with the memory of this place. One possible driver for this is the stress hormone cortisol, which increases steadily across the night. High cortisol concentrations can block communication between the hippocampus and neocortex, and since concentrations are much higher early in the morning, this could provide a physiological reason for the disjointed properties of late-night (early morning) dreams.

Irrespective of how it happens, it is clear that dreams not only replay memory fragments but also create brand-new, highly creative mixtures of memories and knowledge. This process has led to the creation of many works of literature, art, and science, such as Mary Shelley's *Frankenstein,* the molecular formula of benzene, and the invention of the light bulb. An especially good demonstration of this somnolent creativity comes from a study of 35 professional musicians who not only heard more music in their dreams than your normal man-on-the-street but also reported that much of this (28 percent) was music they had never heard in waking life. They had created new music in their dreams!

Although we don't quite understand how dreams achieve this type of innovative recombination of material, it seems clear that the sleeping brain is somehow freed of constraints and can thus create whole sequences of free associations. This is not only useful for creativity, it is also thought to facilitate insight and problem solving. It may even be critical for the integration of newly acquired memories with more remote ones (see chapter 8). In fact, this facilitated lateral thinking could, in itself, be the true purpose of dreams. It is certainly valuable enough to have evolved through natural selection.

FORGETTING OF DREAMS

Even if dreams serve a vital function, and even if they *are* important for memory consolidation, most still seem to fade from memory very soon after waking up. In fact, there is probably a physiological reason that we forget our dreams. When we are awake, the hippocampus monitors activity in the neocortex, keeping track of all the major neural events that happen there, binding together their elements and (most critically) remembering them. When we sleep, however, this pattern changes because the hippocampus becomes much less responsive to inputs from the neocortex. This means that the cortical activity isn't being recorded in the same way as it would be during wake, so the episodes, themes, and stories created in our dreams are not captured. Thus, the same physiological disconnect which makes us construct bizarre combinations and sequences of events when we dream also tends to keep us from remembering them later on when we are awake. If you think about it, this disconnect is probably adaptive since it could be confusing if we remembered our dreams so well that we mixed them up with reality.

Of course, this intentional amnesia for dreams doesn't always work. If it did you wouldn't be reading a chapter about dreams because we wouldn't know they existed. It is unclear why dream amnesia is only partial, but this incomplete pattern suggests that communication between the hippocampus and neocortex is not entirely cut off during sleep—it is just slowed or downgraded (think about a slow Internet connection), so some of the stronger stimuli occurring in the neocortex will still eventually make it into the hippocampus and be remembered. Reduced connectivity of this type could also explain why the dreams we remember are often emotional: Emotional stimuli are stronger, and so perhaps this helps them to penetrate even when there is limited connectivity.

DREAMS AS MEMORY REPLAY?

Another possible mechanism for the preferential remembering of emotional dreams relates to memory replay. The idea that dreams may be a conscious manifestation of the same spontaneous replaying of memories which underpins consolidation during sleep is just too tantalizing to neglect. Although it is unlikely that every single memory replay could surface in this manner, it is possible that a small percentage of replays (the tip of the iceberg) do. Researchers have tested this idea by checking for a relationship between the dreams people report having and the memories which improve during that same epoch of sleep. Specifically, they have looked to see whether people who report dreaming about a newly learned task (like exploring a maze, for instance) improve more across sleep than people who make no such reports.[13] Although it is still relatively early days for this idea, the existing data provide fairly consistent support. One problem with these studies is that because people forget their dreams, researchers have to test vast numbers in order to get a decent sample of "rememberers." The latest wave of experiments have tried to get around this by making the to-be-remembered tasks as emotive as possible. For example, instead of running around fairly mundane 3D mazes on a computer as in older studies, people participating in these experiments are immersed in interactive video game scenarios in which they are racing a clock for survival, and bogeymen may jump out at any corner of the maze while the participants' potential monetary reward visibly dwindles in one corner of the computer screen. This has led to a greater degree of dream incorporation (and memory), but the jury is still out on how these relate to subsequent memory.

SUMMING UP

This chapter has introduced dreams as physical responses which are linked to specific patterns of brain activity. We mentioned the idea that dreams are epiphenomena that result from the random neural firing in the cortex triggered by disordered activity in the brainstem, as well as the idea that dreams are generated by more thinking parts of the brain such as the anterior cingulate. We saw that lesions to the ventromedial prefrontal cortex abolish dreaming, possibly because the dopaminergic reward system which projects through this region is essential for generating dreams. We also explored some potential functions of dreaming, touching on threat simulation and mood regulation, as well as memory replay. Focusing more specifically on memory, we saw that there is a period several days after learning when memories are less likely to be incorporated in dreams, and this is thought to reflect a gradual consolidation process which renders memories temporarily unavailable. Finally, we reviewed the possibility that dreams are important for memory consolidation because they reflect memory replay, and we saw that while memories are sometimes replayed in a more complete form early in the night, only fragments are replayed later in the night, perhaps reflecting the limited connectivity between the hippocampus and neocortex at this time.

The next chapter will take a different angle on consolidation by considering how sleep helps us to abstract overall principles or "gist" from a corpus of information, thus facilitating the construction of general knowledge, as well as creative connections and inferences.

eight

sleep, semantics, and the mind

OLD WIVES' TALES TELL US THAT when we don't understand something, have a hard decision to make, or are upset, we should sleep on it, and much of the difficulty will fade away. Though this ultra-passive advice may have been annoying when we received it as adolescents, most of us have subsequently learned the value of sleep as a time-tested strategy for solving problems. Cuddling down under the covers certainly feels more like a form of evasion than a proactive approach, but sleeping may actually turn out to be one of the most proactive ways you could possibly try to solve whatever problem is bothering you.

Let us tackle this issue bit by bit. Even though we are not consciously thinking about our conundrums while asleep, there is ample evidence that our brains are working on them nevertheless. We saw in chapter 1 that simple skills, like pressing buttons in a specific sequence or riding a bicycle, improve after sleep. More standard examples of memory—such as the recollection of what you had for breakfast, what you did yesterday, or (experimentally) the memory of a set of pictures or words you have been shown—are also retained better over time spent asleep than over the same amount of time spent awake. Even brief naps, some as short as six minutes, can benefit memory. Sleep clearly does something to memories, and the fact that some types of memory are actually *stronger* after sleep suggests we are not just talking about passive protection against decay or interference (i.e., preventing memories from crumbling, or from being overwritten by, or confused with, other incoming information). Instead, sleep appears to actively process memories in a way that noticeably strengthens them. This is old news to anyone who read chapters 5 and 7, as you will know that background noise which might have interfered with memories is routinely cleared away during sleep, and also that memories are replayed during sleep in a way that leads to a specific strengthening of representations.

However, the fact that memories are actively strengthened while we snooze doesn't explain why we gradually come to respect our mothers' uninspiring advice to "sleep on it" as a way of solving our trickiest dilemmas. Why should having stronger memories for individual events make our problems any easier to solve? The answer appears to be that sleep does a lot more than just strengthen individual memories. It is also involved in the complex process of integrating new information with old and in abstracting out the general principles or rules which describe a corpus of events and help us to make informed predictions about the future.

For instance, after attending a number of children's birthday parties, you will gradually figure out that these events almost invariably involve some kind of a cake, presents, and lots of (hopefully happy) children. Other characteristics of the parties, such as the presence of helium balloons, clowns, specific people, and the place where the party is held, may vary hugely from one occasion to another, but the more constant characteristics should provide a framework which lets you form a mental representation of what a birthday party is like. Once you have this basic representation, you can more easily attach information about the less frequent properties (e.g., some birthday parties are held at a swimming pool) together with an idea of how likely this is (maybe about 10 percent of the parties in your town are held at a pool) and what other characteristics go along with them (when they are held at a pool, there's a 75 percent chance there will be watermelon). This representation of the core characteristics of a party, how likely these are to occur, and which characteristics go together make it much easier for you to make predictions about future parties—and in some cases to deal with tricky decisions about whether to take sunscreen, what type of gift to purchase, and so forth.

There's growing evidence that sleep helps us to create the type of unified representation that I've described. Because the creation of such a representation is pretty complex, formal studies tend to break it down into specific steps. For instance, some experiments have looked at the role of sleep in integrating disparate fragments of information into a unified whole. Other studies have looked at how sleep promotes the integration of new learning with older knowledge, and some particularly ambitious researchers have even argued that sleep facilitates creativity and insight because it helps to form connections between distantly related ideas or concepts (such as realizing that people who live in temperate climates are more likely to have pool parties if their birthday is in the summer, while people who live in the tropics may have such parties year-round). Studies which more specifically target the formation of cognitive frameworks have examined sleep's role in the extraction of specific aspects of a situation which are repeated in many memories (presents, cake, happy children) to form a basic knowledge framework, which we will refer to as a schema. Scientifically, we tend to refer to this process of distilling out the shared characteristics as "abstraction." The cognitive frameworks (or schemas) which are abstracted in this way allow us to structure our knowledge and make valid predictions about the future (such as that relating to birthday parties). How could sleep possibly influence the construction of such schemas? Let's take a closer look.

Perhaps the clearest support for the idea that sleep facilitates the binding together of individual memories in a way that lets you see the bigger picture comes from a study using something called transitive inference.[1] In this study, the experimenters arbitrarily labeled a set of abstract pictures as A, B, C, D, E, and F. Due to these labels (and nothing else) the pictures fell into a hierarchy: A > B > C > D > E > F. However, the people participating in the experiment were told about neither the labels nor the hierarchy. As far as they could see there was no special relationship between the pictures, except that they were presented

in pairs, with one always being indicated as > (greater than) than
the other (e.g., A > B, B > C, C > D, D > E, and E > F). All these
pairs involved adjacent pictures, so even if they were all remembered, the people participating in the study would have to make
a sort of cognitive leap to realize that B > D, or C > F, for example. However, after training, people were tested on exactly these
types of inferences, and the results showed that they could make
these leaps much more successfully after they had slept than after they had spent an equal amount of time awake. It looked as
though the sleep somehow helped them to integrate the fragments and create a unified representation of everything they had
learned about these pictures, and how they all fit together.

A study of insight in problem solving provides further evidence that sleep supports the extraction of common themes from
repeated experiences.[2] Participants in this study were asked to
solve a mathematical problem through repetition of the same rule
again and again as they recursively solved a series of nested equations to get to a final solution. What they weren't told was that
the answer to the second recursive equation was also always the
answer to the overall problem (Fig. 21). Once they realized this,

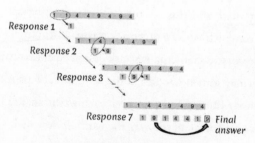

Fig. 21   The number reduction task

it was possible to avoid working through the bulk of the recursive equations and instead jump straight to the final solution. After a night of sleep, about half of the group was faster at solving recursive equations. The other half was no faster, but fascinatingly it was this slow cohort that tended to deduce the rule, and therefore eventually to improve their overall speed more dramatically than they could have done by quick performance of the dreary recursive solving. Through an insight into the overall structure of the problem, this group was able to skip to the final answer after solving just the first two equations. The really interesting thing here is not just the fact that people got better at this task, but that they got better in two different ways—either they solved the recursive problems faster, or they integrated all the information they had about the task and worked out that there was a shortcut. These two processes seem to be mutually exclusive since only the slow group tended to find the shortcut.

A related experiment examined the impact of sleep on creativity by asking people to solve word puzzles.[3] Three words, for instance, *sixteen, heart,* and *tooth,* were shown, and people had to figure out which fourth word linked them all together (in this case, *sweet* would be a good answer). People were significantly better at coming up with the answers to this type of problem after a 90-minute nap, and this advantage was only apparent in people who got some REM sleep during that nap. Taken in combination with the recursive mathematical task described above, this suggests that sleep may somehow assist in the formation of associations between loosely interrelated concepts, such as the shared pattern in the math problems and the way the word *sweet* associates with all three cue words (sweet-tooth, sweet-heart, sweet-sixteen).

Even clearer support for the idea that sleep allows this type of integrative thinking comes from studies which search directly for evidence that snoozing plays a role in pulling together loosely related bits of information.[4] For instance, people were taught the meanings of a series of Japanese characters, each of which contained a small pictorial component called a radical, which indicated that it belonged to a particular conceptual category. They were then shown a new (unlearned) character, which contained the same radical, and asked to select one of four possible meanings for it (Fig. 22). Finally people were shown the radical in isolation and asked to type its meaning. Because the radicals were never pointed out in the original characters, this task required integration across multiple pieces of information (e.g., the various characters that pertain to a category, such as *water*) and abstraction of the information which is common to all of them (this particular bit of the character that is shared indicates membership in the category *water*). People did much better on this complex abstraction task after sleep.

More abstract examples of the same general principle come from tasks in which people are asked to extract general statistics from a set of information arranged according to probabilistic

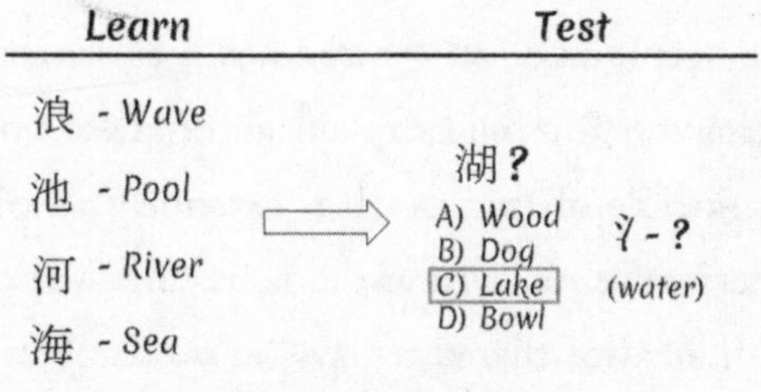

Learn	Test
浪 - *Wave*	
池 - *Pool*	湖 **?**
⟹	A) Wood
河 - *River*	B) Dog
	C) Lake 氵 - **?**
海 - *Sea*	D) Bowl (water)

Fig. 22   Japanese character task

rules.[5] For instance, if participants had been exposed to a continuous stream of auditory tones which were organized probabilistically (tone A was followed by tone B with a 90 percent probability, tone B was followed by tone C with a 90 percent probability, and so forth) for a few minutes, they were subsequently better able to differentiate short snippets of tone sequence which conformed to the same probabilistically determined pattern from randomly ordered snippets after a night of sleep. In fact, their ability to recognize structured sequences improved significantly overnight.

Taken together, these studies demonstrate that sleep is important for combining information from multiple sources. It helps us to extract statistical regularities, pull out general principles, integrate newly formed memories with older knowledge structures, and piece together a larger picture from a set of interrelated fragments. But how does sleep facilitate these processes? This problem remains to be solved, but there is at least one promising potential explanation.

In 2011, with my colleague Simon Durrant, now at the University of Lincoln, I developed a model called information overlap to abstract (iOtA), which attempts to explain how replaying memories during slow wave sleep, in combination with the downscaling of connections between neurons which also occurs in that sleep phase (otherwise known as synaptic homeostasis, see chapter 5), could explain all of these phenomena.[6] The basic principle of this model is extremely simple: If more than one memory is replayed at the same time, the neurons associated with areas of shared replay, or "overlap," will be more strongly activated than the other neurons (Fig. 23). This means,

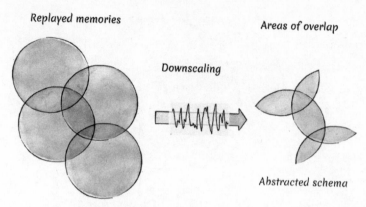

Fig. 23   The information overlap to abstract (iOtA) model

for instance, if you replay memories of two or three different birthday parties, all of which involved cake, presents, and balloons, but each of which was held in a different place and with a different set of guests, then responses in the neurons which code for cake, presents, and balloons will be stronger than responses associated with the locations of individual parties or the people who attended them. Furthermore, based on the general principle that neurons which fire together wire together (see chapter 3), the linkages between neural representations of cake, presents, and balloons will also become stronger than other linkages associated with these memories, such as between a specific birthday girl and her presents or the other people who were at her party (Fig. 24). All of this strengthening is important because it means that when the synapses are subsequently downscaled these representations of overlap may be the only thing that is retained. In fact, as multiple memories are replayed across a night, the more often a specific representation (say, a birthday cake) or pair

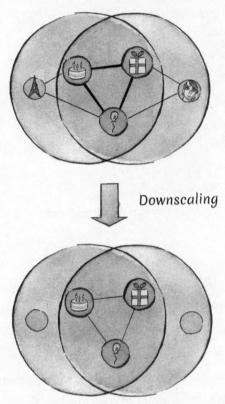

Downscaling

Fig. 24   Only shared memory components survive downscaling

of representations (say, both cake and presents) is triggered, the more likely that specific aspect of a memory is to be retained.

How does the iOtA model explain the data on integration and problem solving which I described above? Well, it makes quick work of the Japanese symbols task since this requires people to learn that a specific radical is always associated with a specific concept (e.g., female in the example above). If the memory representations of several different characters are replayed concurrently during slow wave sleep, they will all trigger responses in both the radical and the representation of female, so these will become strongly activated and will bind together. If this happens enough, the association will be retained even when representations of the individual characters are lost. The same is true for the calculation task: Because the shortcut rule works for every single calculation problem, replaying just a few of these would invariably strengthen that commonality. The transitive inference task, with the hierarchy A > B > C, etc., can be explained through the construction of a series of associations that gradually builds up to provide the full hierarchy. This means individual pairs like B > C are no longer perceived as individual because B is linked to A, and C is linked to D, which is linked to E, and so forth. The statistical learning task provides slightly more of a challenge for the iOtA model. To learn the statistical properties of a task, we don't just need to remember simple associations—we need to learn *how likely* it is that those associations will occur. This means the brain would need to keep track of how often one tone is followed by another—such as tone A followed by tone B—by averaging across the various replays of these memories. Although the iOtA model doesn't currently explain how this type of averaging occurs, it isn't difficult to see how it *could occur.*

Although the ability of sleep, and specifically overlapping memory replay during sleep, to produce these results is impressive, there is also a deeper subtext here.

The realization that birthday parties are associated with cake, presents, and balloons is an example of the development of new semantic, or conceptual, knowledge. Semantic knowledge is the general knowledge about the world and how things in it relate to each other. Classic examples of semantic knowledge are knowledge that the sky is blue, that Paris is the capital of France, and for that matter that birthday parties normally include cake, presents, and balloons. Fascinatingly, although we all have such knowledge, we can never remember where we learned it. In fact, remembering the origin of such knowledge actually disqualifies it from being considered to be semantic. People with certain forms of brain damage or atrophy such as semantic dementia have deteriorations in semantic knowledge which, if severe enough, can be catastrophic for their daily lives. For a start, such impairments commonly make it hard to find the words they need to express themselves. Worse still, semantic dementia patients may be easily confused and have trouble carrying out even simple activities like making a cup of tea (they might, for example, forget to boil the water, forget to use a tea bag, or muddle things up by boiling the milk or using salt instead of sugar).

Although semantic knowledge is essential for everything we do, scientists don't know much about how it is formed. General theories of memory suggest that representations of individual experiences evolve over time and, through a process of repeated replay in the neocortex, gradually become integrated with the knowledge you already have. The iOtA model extends these theories by showing how memory replay during sleep could form the building blocks of semantic memories, as well as helping new memories to integrate with the knowledge which already exists.

SUMMING UP

Does sleeping on a complex problem really help us to solve it? The type of integration and abstraction which we've discussed here, and which can be explained by the iOtA model, may not help with every single problem you ever encounter in your life—but it would normally be worth at least giving it a chance (e.g. by getting a night or two of sleep) before you decide the issue is insoluble. These ideas provide an initial understanding of why we gradually come to respect our mothers when they tell us to "sleep on it"—but the precise mechanism by which this overnight memory magic occurs remains to be explored.

nine

emotional memories and sleep

ALL MEMORIES ARE NOT CREATED
equal. We remember emotionally loaded events much better
than everyday happenings. This makes a lot of sense from an
evolutionary perspective since the things we feel strongly about
are normally a lot more important than everything else. Being kissed by someone we're attracted to, getting ill after eating a particular mushroom, or the name of that amazing ice
cream your friend gave you are all examples of things which
it would probably be a good idea to remember. On the other
hand, many aspects of the daily grind—such as what you had
for breakfast, where you put your keys, or where you parked
your bicycle seem much less important (although this may not
turn out to be the case if you can't eventually find the keys or
bicycle).

It is no accident that emotional memories are remembered better than anything else. In fact, evolutionary psychologists would argue that emotion only exists as a mechanism for flagging important events to ensure they are given preferential treatment by your memory-generation mechanisms thereafter and are thus more likely to be strongly coded and retained. Cavemen who didn't preferentially remember which foods were okay to give to a baby, which hunting techniques lead to a successful kill, and where the tigers tended to hang out probably didn't survive too long. It is really essential that important information is remembered, and emotions are markers of what's important. The way the body and brain respond to an emotion influences the way events are recorded in our memories at the outset, as well as the gradual changes in such memories as they evolve across time.

EMOTION AND THE AMYGDALA

One of the first brain areas to react to an incoming emotion is an almond-shaped structure called the amygdala. You have two amygdalas, one in each hemisphere of your brain, and these are tucked away somewhere around the front of your ears, just a few centimeters below the scalp. Neurons in these structures fire strongly in response to threatening or unpleasant stimuli (like the scary pictures or nasty electric shocks which scientists like to give people when they study negative or fearful emotions). The amygdala response is very quick—in fact it occurs well before you are aware of whatever's scaring you—and often irrespective of whether or not you are paying attention to it. Neurons in

the amygdala connect back to sensory areas in the brain, for instance, those involved in processing visual, auditory, and tactile
information (as well as to lots of other places); the fast response
means the amygdala can "turn up the volume" in these areas,
allowing stronger and more accurate sensory detection of whatever is threatening.

Sensory structures aren't the only places where the amygdalas influence neural activity. They also project to the hippocampus, which you will remember is absolutely central to forming
new memories. It still isn't clear exactly how the nudging of the
hippocampus by the amygdala could lead to stronger memory
representations, but it is pretty clear that's what happens. For
instance, if the neural connection from amygdala to hippocampus is blocked (something that most commonly occurs when
a callous scientist administers drugs that clog up the receptors
which mediate communication between these structures), emotional memories lose their edge—they are remembered only as
well as run of the mill everyday memories. This could mean, for
example, that you remembered your first kiss only as well as the
first time you did something fairly mundane, like eating tuna
fish or putting on a specific pair of unexciting shoes.

If your amygdalas get damaged, or behave abnormally,
there are lots of potential side effects. For instance, if these little
neural almonds don't respond to dangerous situations you may
wind up taking much bigger risks than you would otherwise
have done. Some good examples of this come from extreme
thrill seekers—BASE jumpers (those daredevils who jump off
cliffs or tall buildings with a parachute), extreme skiers, and the

like. Comparisons between the brains of these nutters and the rest of us less cavalier mortals have shown that, in such habitual risk-takers, the amygdala response is highly abnormal. The neurons don't increase their firing rates as they would in the average couch potato who finds himself in a risky environment. Instead, other areas of the brain which are associated with pleasure and reward are sometimes engaged. These neural responses provide physiological evidence of what you might think is obvious: Such daredevil sportsmen are not only fearless (i.e., lacking the amygdala response) but they also get a kick out of danger (engagement of reward-related areas). If these data are reliable (and that is quite a big *if* since this has only been studied in a few BASE jumpers), they go a long way toward explaining why these guys head back to the tops of their cliffs, waterfalls, and ski-jumps again and again, even if they have been injured or had bad experiences there.

Another common side effect of amygdala damage is the inability to recognize emotion in other people's facial expressions. Fearful and threatening expressions are the trickiest for patients with this type of issue. This might not sound like a huge problem, but these cues are actually pretty important for your interactions with other people. If someone is threatening you, for instance, it is certainly good for you to know about it. Likewise, if something happens that scares the people around you, it would probably be a good idea for you to realize they are scared, especially if you also have a reduced response to fear yourself. The clues you get from other people might be the only thing which saves you from becoming a tasty (or stringy, depending on your BMI) dinner!

CONSOLIDATION AND EMOTIONAL MEMORY

Of course, memory isn't really about making a permanent, fixed record of things that happen. Scary as it sounds, memories are flexible, malleable, and evolve over time. What's special about emotional memories is that any advantage they have over more mundane representations gets stronger as time passes.

It is pretty clear, at least in people with a healthy fear of BASE jumping, that the amygdala is involved in this preferential trajectory of emotional memories and doesn't merely control how they are coded into the brain at the outset. Evidence comes from studies which show that manipulating amygdala responses after the fact can alter how well the event is remembered later on. For example, injecting something to excite or inhibit amygdala activity about ten minutes after your first kiss could prevent that memory from achieving the special status it should normally have as a strongly emotional memory. Sadly enough, if the connection between amygdala and hippocampus is blocked immediately after this highly emotional memory is formed, it will be forgotten at the same rate as a mundane, everyday memory (think again of your initial experiences of tuna fish or putting on those rather boring shoes). This system is useful because it means the emotional reaction you have after the experience has a chance to influence how well you remember it. Thinking back to the cavemen, it should be obvious why the tasty meal which follows a successful hunting trip would influence how well the strategies used to bring down the prey are remembered. Once an emotional memory of this type has been formed, it isn't clear if it can easily be overwritten. So you may remember that new hunting technique for time immemorial, even if it never works again. On the other hand, if you subsequently have a lot of bad experiences with that technique, this memory may gradually become associated with failure rather than success.

It is this point about the consolidation, or evolution, of a memory—between when you first encode it and when you next try to call it back—that brings us again to the topic of sleep. Emotionally laden memories aren't just better remembered than their neutral counterparts; they are also more strongly protected by sleep. This doesn't necessarily mean they are stronger after you've slept than they were beforehand. It could just mean they are less likely to weaken across sleep. In practice, your memory of that first kiss might be as strong as ever ten years after it happened, but the initially comparable memory of your early experiences with tuna fish has probably been lost completely.

This preferential strengthening or protection of emotional memories is what scientists think of as a fragile effect. That means, disappointingly enough, in a very frustrating (but hopefully small) proportion of experiments, we don't find any preferential strengthening at all. In other (still frustrating) experiments, preferential strengthening is only apparent in weaker memories possibly because stronger ones will probably be retained even if they aren't strengthened during consolidation. When the effect is there, however, the advantage to emotional memories is persistent: Even four years after the event, tests show a marked superiority of negative memories in people who were allowed to sleep after reading an upsetting story about child murder compared to those who were kept awake.[1]

So what happens during sleep that specifically protects emotional memories? The real answer is, we don't know. It is reasonable to expect that emotional memories are reactivated and replayed during sleep just like neutral memories, and this replay helps to preferentially strengthen them by changing the way they are coded in the brain. Plenty of clues suggest that REM sleep is important for this process. For a start, the REM-rich sleep we get during the last part of the night seems to lead to preferential consolidation of emotional memories. The sleep we get earlier in the night, which contains little REM, doesn't seem to be important for this. Furthermore, during REM sleep it is quite common to find whole populations of neurons that fire at a specific frequency (called theta-band) of 4 to 8 Hz. The extent to which such neural activity is observed in a particular REM episode can predict the extent to which emotional memories will be strengthened, so more theta-band activity seems to mean more emotional-specific strengthening. Interestingly, the amygdala and hippocampus both go more or less crazy in REM sleep, with much higher levels of neural firing than would normally be observed during wake. Furthermore, the frequency of some of this frenetic activity (the theta-band oscillations) is phase-locked, meaning neurons in the amygdala and hippocampus are firing at essentially the same time, in a way that is only ever seen in the awake brain during really arousing experiences. It is difficult to know exactly what this means, but most neuroscientists would agree that coordinated firing in two tightly interconnected brain structures is a sign that they are working together. We know the amygdala and hippocampus work together both when an emotional event is being stored away in the hippocampus (as in those really arousing wakeful experiences mentioned above) and when you're trying to remember it later on, so the fact that they are also in communication during REM sleep suggests that these structures are somehow working on or processing the neural representations of these memories while you sleep. Although the research has yet to be conducted, I would hazard a guess that this tight communication between amygdala and hippocampus occurs when emotional memories are replayed in REM and is somehow essential for processing feelings. The heightened communication between these structures should allow such memories to be preferentially strengthened, often resulting in the stronger amygdala responses, greater connectivity, and more successful recollection, which is often observed when emotional material is remembered after sleep.

SUPPRESSING MUNDANE MEMORIES?

Sleep's preferential treatment of emotional memories isn't limited to a simple strengthening or protection of things that are important. There is evidence that sleep practices an active form of discrimination, strengthening some memories and neglecting, or even actively suppressing, others. Under this line of thinking the neural processing which occurs in sleep mediates a trade-off between emotional memories and memories that are less important or attention grabbing. Imagine, for instance, that you are being mugged by an armed robber. Some aspects of what you see will be really important—like the gun in his hand, the way he points it at you, the escape route you find, and so forth. You will probably remember these things. Other details, like the color of surrounding buildings, the background sounds, the type of tree you are standing under, or who passes by in the distance, may seem less important. You are less likely to carve out space in your hippocampus for these details in the first place. This—the fact that you remember the most important or salient items in a scene, and forget (or maybe don't even notice) less important details—is known as the "weapon focus effect."

In an early study of the weapon focus effect two groups of participants attended what they thought was going to be a regular experiment on memory. In fact, it was a fairly dramatic simulation. Volunteers in one condition sat in a waiting room where they overheard a heated discussion, then saw a man leaving with a grease pencil. In the other condition volunteers sat in the same waiting room, but instead of a discussion, they heard furniture being thrown around as part of a violent argument and then saw a man leave holding a blood-stained letter opener. During a subsequent photo line-up, volunteers who had seen the grease pencil were more likely to accurately identify a man who was holding it than participants who saw the letter opener (49 percent versus 33 percent correct identifications).[2]

The really interesting thing about the weapon focus isn't that people remember details about the weapon—that is pretty much to be expected—it is that they tend to remember other details less well than they would have if no weapon had been present. This is due to a limitation on resources—we can't attend to everything in a situation, and we can't consolidate and retain everything we have seen. If something is really important we invest a larger share of the total resources we have on offer in it, so the stuff that was less important is less likely to be remembered.

Fascinatingly, it looks as though sleep facilitates this trade-off. Studies of emotional memories which contain both an attention-grabbing central element and more mundane peripheral elements (e.g., a photograph of a car crash on a regular suburban street) show that sleep enhances the trade-off. After people sleep they not only remember the car crash better, they are also less likely to recognize the background street. It looks as though sleep, while working to cement memories that are really important, may also need to pare down the less important ones, clearing up space and resources for what matters. One way of thinking about this paring away of unimportant memories relates to the synaptic homeostasis hypothesis described in chapter 5. Synaptic downscaling during sleep is not just a physical lessening of connections; it very likely also represents the pruning of unwanted memories—presumably, mundane memories about the background in which a nasty car crash occurred fall into this category. So the dramatic reduction in synapses which occurs in slow wave sleep should be associated with a parallel reduction of the types of useless memories that normally create noise in the radio signal of our recollection.

INTENTIONALITY AND SLEEP

Emotion isn't the only thing which can determine whether a memory is strengthened or weakened by sleep. Simply believing that something is important (for instance, being warned that you'll be tested on it the next day) seems to have a big effect on the kind of consolidation that happens during sleep. One study examined this by asking people to learn two sets of information such as two lists of word pairs on different occasions. On one occasion they were told they would be tested the next day on what they learned, and on the other occasion they were not. Of course, they were actually tested on all the information on both occasions, but overnight improvements in performance were only observed for items on which they expected a post-sleep test. The participants' memories not only improved selectively when they had been told the material they learned would be tested; characteristics of their sleep, e.g., the amount of slow oscillations and sleep spindles (those high-frequency 10–15 Hz waves of activity that we compared to children jumping into a lake and briefly thrashing around in chapter 1) they had between initial learning and the subsequent test predicted this improvement. Conversely, sleep patterns in the control group bore no relation to subsequent memory performance. This little trick, called retrieval expectancy, worked for several types of memory, including finger tapping and object location memories.[3] Another study showed very similar effects when volunteers were told to either remember or forget individual words. A 90-minute nap led to facilitated memory for only the "remember" words, and this was predicted by the sleep spindles obtained.[4]

   In general, it appears that consolidation processes, including sleep, selectively target information which seems important. Importance can be determined cognitively by the person who is trying to remember since it can be influenced by both emotionality of the to-be-remembered material and simple knowledge that the information is important or will be used later.

REM, DEPRESSION, AND EMOTIONAL MEMORY

Interestingly (and perhaps unhappily), people who suffer from depression tend to have more REM sleep than would be considered normal. Negative memories are the ones that seem to be really protected by REM. There isn't much work on positive memories, but what is there hasn't shown a big protective effect. So if sleep does selectively preserve positive memories against decay then it doesn't seem to do this to such a great extent as it does for negative memories. Is it possible that excessive REM could be making depression worse—or at least keeping people in a low-mood cycle by selectively boosting memory of all of the bad things that happened to them, while more happy (or at least neutral) thoughts are allowed to wither away to nothing?

Many antidepressant drugs suppress REM—and this could be one potential mechanism through which they help to combat depression. These drugs are typically SSRIs (selective serotonin reuptake inhibitors), which do just what their name says: They prevent serotonin from being collected out of the synapse and parceled away into storage. The ultimate impact of an SSRI is to increase the amount of serotonin available in the synapse. Serotonin, of course, is a "feel good" neurotransmitter, so having it around in increased concentrations leads to a better mood. The increased serotonin also blocks REM since it inhibits the "REM-on" cells that trigger this sleep state (see chapter 4).

In fact, REM sleep reproduces some of the brain imbalances associated with major depressive disorder. In depression, the limbic system and ventromedial prefrontal cortex are overactive, while the dorsolateral prefrontal cortex, which normally regulates responses in those areas, is suppressed. This pattern has the characteristics of a self-reinforcing cycle since the abnormally strong negative responses in the amygdala and ventromedial prefrontal cortex can't be inhibited via cognitive strategies which are implemented by the dorsolateral prefrontal cortex (e.g., reevaluation of circumstances). One study, which looked directly at this top-down connection between dorsolateral prefrontal cortex and amygdala, showed that sleep deprivation essentially cut the connection between these structures, leading to excessive amygdala responses when people saw nasty pictures.[5] While the cortical areas were apparently able to keep the amygdala somewhat in check when well rested, sleep deprivation seemed to impair this ability to regulate that wayward little structure. Of course, this doesn't show that sleep is part of the problem in depression—instead it merely provides a tantalizing hint about sleep's role in the regulation of emotions by telling us that abnormalities in sleep could change this important inhibitory connection in a way that could potentially lead to depression.

In addition to strengthening negative memories, REM sleep is also thought to recalibrate emotional responses which get distorted across a day of wakefulness. Studies investigating this have used photos of faces expressing a range of emotions (happy, fearful, sad, disgusted, and angry). People react in an excessively negative way to faces that have just a hint of an angry and fearful expression after a day of normal wakeful activity, but getting a bit of REM sleep reverses this effect.[6] Also, when REM is increased in depression, slow wave sleep is normally decreased, leading to a state of chronic slow wave deprivation. This might not sound too important until you think about how you felt last time you were seriously sleep deprived. The answer should be "not that good" (or worse). Studies of how people feel after sleep deprivation show increased irritability and a more negative outlook, which causes amplification of neural responses to aversive events and a blunting of responses to happy events. More subtle bodily responses are also influenced by sleep deprivation; for instance, the pupil dilation response to happy or sad pictures is larger, suggesting a failure of regulation.

All of this has been taken as evidence that sleep is needed to reset a system of emotional responses which is regulated by the dorsolateral and medial prefrontal cortices. This pattern of disregulation has also been observed in depression and other psychiatric disorders which feature alterations in sleep patterns. Although this proposed causal relationship between increased REM and decreased slow wave sleep in depression has yet to be firmly established, the very idea of it is exciting to psychiatrists, since sleep is something of an unexplored frontier when it comes to treatment for mood disorders.

SUMMING UP

This chapter has explained that sleep strengthens emotional memories even more than neutral ones. REM sleep, with its high-frequency theta-band oscillations, seems to be particularly important for this, and the overstrengthening of negative memories may cause problems in depression since depressed people get more than the usual quota of REM. It is possible that the overstrengthening of negative memories during REM contributes to making people depressed and keeping them that way. Many effective antidepressant drugs actually suppress REM, which could mean that they partially fight depression by preventing pernicious overconsolidation of the negative. Sleep also recalibrates emotional responses, which seem to get more negative as we become more and more tired during the day. This will be old news to anyone who is aware of their own grumpiness late in the evening!

In general, sleep seems to be working hard to make sure we keep hold of the most important memories and respond appropriately to stimuli we come across during the day. But how does sleep affect the way we actually feel about emotional events that have happened to us? The next chapter will take a detailed look at this and also explain why it is a highly controversial topic.

ten

does sleep disarm
dangerous emotions?

IMAGINE YOU WITNESSED A TERRIBLE accident earlier today. Two cars slammed into each other just ahead of you on the motorway—and nobody got out. You rushed to help and managed to extract a little girl from the back seat of one car, but she was unconscious and bleeding. You did everything you could, but when the paramedics finally got there, they said it was no use—she had died in your arms. This was a scarring experience, which left horrendous images in your mind that just won't go away. You've talked to a few friends, and they calmed you down a bit, but all the conversations finished with useless suggestions like, "Get some rest and you'll feel better." Are you really going to feel better about this horrific event after a night of sleep? One of the new theories in the study of sleep and memory suggests that you will. The overnight therapy hypothesis suggests that active processing during REM sleep causes negative memories to lose their bite.[1] We are all familiar with the idea of feeling better in the morning, but is it really true, and could it work for these horrible images you have of the crash?

Let's back away for a minute and take a broader look at how emotions work in the brain. Once this is clear we will evaluate evidence for and against the concept of overnight therapy.

The almond-like amygdala located deep in the temporal lobe of your brain can, very loosely, be thought of as a fear detector (although it also responds to other emotions such as anger and even happiness). It reacts very quickly to emotional situations, drastically increasing neural firing rates as soon as you experience something scary or upsetting. Although this little structure has a massive influence on what happens next, in terms of physiological responses, it isn't the only part of the body which reacts early. When you're really frightened by an outside stimulus, many bodily systems engage quickly in preparation for fast action. This is often called the "fight or flight" response because it gets you ready for action, whether by fleeing the scene or standing up to the danger. Blood is pumped from the skin and organs to the muscles, priming them for movement; pupils dilate, presumably to allow more light in; the heart pounds and hairs can stand on end; and the interesting thing is that all of this happens before you are even aware of the emotion.

There is evidence that you don't actually feel afraid (happy, sad, etc.) until your brain has picked up on these various bodily responses and interpreted them. If this is correct, then emotion actually results directly from a sort of read-out of the body's state.[2] A really fascinating perspective on this is the idea that nothing can feel scary if the body doesn't respond to it. That might sound strange, but this idea is precisely what forms the basis of the overnight therapy hypothesis.

So how could overnight therapy work? The increased heart rate, clenched teeth, tightened buttocks—whatever you consider as part of the unconscious bodily response to fear—is largely controlled by a neurotransmitter called norepinephrine. Without norepinephrine your body just wouldn't have those terror-inspiring responses even in the scariest situations. And here's the trick: Brain levels of norepinephrine reach an all-time low during REM sleep. So, if memories are replayed during REM, then no matter how scary they are, they won't be associated with the normal bodily response because there simply isn't enough norepinephrine around to elicit these. In other words, when you're in REM sleep and dreaming of a frightening event, your emotional system cannot respond normally. The overnight therapy hypothesis proposes that, even though the content of the memory may be strengthened through this type of emotion-free replay, its emotionality could be completely lost (if it is replayed often enough, that is).

Overnight therapy is attractive as an idea not just because of its conceptual tidiness but also because of vast bodies of anecdotal evidence. We have all experienced the therapeutic effects of a night of sleep when we are upset, and we all know it is often better to "sleep on" a disagreement before coming back to it. Sleep undoubtedly helps to soothe frayed nerves, calm tempers, provide perspective, and generally alleviate difficult emotional situations. This might seem like the ideal way to process trau-matic events.

Nevertheless, there is plenty of evidence that emotional memories are often preferentially strengthened during sleep (see chapter 9). Proponents of overnight therapy neatly sidestep this issue by pointing out that upsetting events may indeed be bet-ter remembered after sleep—but they simply won't be associ-ated with the same kind of emotional response postsleep as they would have elicited had they not been processed through sleep. The idea is that emotional content is essentially decoupled from the memory as a result of replay in REM sleep. This theory is supported by a recent study in which volunteers were shown an array of pictures, some of which were deeply disturbing scenes of accidents, surgery, disfigurement, and the like.[3] Some were neu-tral scenes, such as landscapes or pictures of rooms or people at leisure, and some were happy scenes of children playing, kittens or puppies, mouth-watering foods (chocolate cake, ice-cream sundae), or couples kissing. People were asked to rate each im-age for emotional intensity both before and after a night of sleep. Fascinatingly, the results revealed that they felt the exact same images were less emotionally intense when seen again after sleep. Responses of neurons in the amygdala to the pictures were also markedly reduced after sleep, and (perhaps most interestingly) these changes were predicted by the neural firing which occurred at frequencies between 25 and 100 Hz during REM sleep. Be-cause neural firing at this frequency (called gamma-band) is a marker of the concentration of the neurotransmitter noradrena-line, this correlation shows that the less noradrenaline there was in the system during REM sleep, the more the pictures lost their emotional impact. The same ratings of emotion were taken before and after a day of wake and revealed no specific change in how people perceived the pictures.

One really fascinating angle of the overnight therapy idea relates to pathological conditions like posttraumatic stress disorder (PTSD). Soldiers coming back from battle and people who have witnessed horrific accidents are just two of the groups that often suffer from this disorder. The flashbacks they experience can come at any time, they may have trouble sleeping, and the rest they do obtain is often haunted by horrific dreams about their experiences. Simply put, PTSD is the repeated, intrusive remembering of highly arousing (and upsetting) negative memories, and the consequences can ruin marriages, destroy lives, and lead to long-term depression and even suicide. If REM really does serve to dissociate memories of horrific situations from the emotional responses that originally accompanied them then it clearly isn't doing its job properly in people with PTSD. Something has gone wrong with the system.

As mentioned earlier, sometimes the best way to verify a neurological process is to see how people who lack one of the parts of the equation fare. There are people who lack the ability to experience normal REM sleep. This is referred to as disregulated REM sleep, and those individuals are at greater risk of PTSD.[4]

We mentioned that one of the reasons it is good to relive the scary events through dreams during REM is the lowered level of the neurotransmitter norepinephrine. It turns out that higher than normal levels of norepinephrine during REM are linked to high risk for PTSD.[5] This fits into the overnight therapy idea like a perfect puzzle piece since having more norepinephrine in the system means that unconscious bodily responses to emotion (such as a faster pulse or dilated pupils) are not reduced. Abnormally high norepinephrine in REM could therefore prevent the decoupling of emotional content from memories when they are reactivated. But hold on a minute. Are we really debating the question of whether replaying a memory with or without autonomic responses could make a difference to what you remember later? How can merely replaying a memory change it for good, irrespective of whether or not that means removing emotionality? After all, aren't memories reasonably fixed and solid?

RECONSOLIDATION

To answer this question we need to back up and talk about a concept called reconsolidation. Memories evolve across time and sleep. The way they are represented in the brain changes, the way they integrate with other memories and with general knowledge changes, and of course they may also be forgotten. Whether or not we can influence or control this evolution of memory poses a really tantalizing question. Imagine how fantastic it would be if you could shape your memories just as you like them (this might not lead to accurate memory, but at least you could have a good time—after the fact that is—and maybe even boost your self-esteem to boot).

Reconsolidation is the idea that memories become flexible and fragile every time we use them, and as such, it offers a potential mechanism by which we can modify them in a semicontrolled manner. To understand reconsolidation, you almost need to think of memories like library books which get stored away somewhere in the deep, dark depths of your brain for years at a time and don't change much once they're stored (except for a gradual rotting and moldering and also an ever-increasing possibility that you won't be able to find them when they're needed). Other than these minor dangers they are pretty safe while in the book-stacks. Once they are called back and brought out for use, however, these books are vulnerable. Sometimes they are slightly rewritten or scribbled on, sometimes they are grouped with related books before they are put back in storage, and sometimes they are damaged or lost. Reshelving is an active process, and messing this up can be so disastrous that these memories are lost completely—for instance, if you don't have the resources to reshelve them or if you somehow put them in the wrong place. Two components of this analogy—the idea that memories are flexible once they have been retrieved, and the idea that storing them again is active and can be disrupted—capture the essence of reconsolidation.

This phenomenon of memory lability has been studied extensively in rats. If these furry creatures learn an association—for instance, between a beep and an imminent electric shock—they normally remember it for months (so long as they don't hear the beep without the shock too many times, that is). One clever experiment used this type of memory to study reconsolidation.[6] Two groups of rats learned to associate a specific sound, called the CS or "conditioned stimulus," with a shock, called the US or "unconditioned stimulus" (Fig. 25.) The fact that they had learned this properly was obvious because every time they heard the beep they froze in fear of the imminent pain. Anisomycin, a substance that prevents cells from creating the proteins needed for consolidation, was injected into the rats' amygdalas 14 days after initial learning. One group of rats heard the beep again once (but without a shock) about four hours before the injection (top). The other group heard nothing (bottom). Twenty-four hours after the injection, all the rats were tested to see if they remembered that the beep was scary. The rats who hadn't heard it since training were just as scared as ever. Amazingly, however, the rats who had heard the sound before the injection ceased to associate it with the electric shock. They showed no sign of fear when they heard the beep on day 15. This acquired amnesia didn't happen if rats were not injected with anisomycin, so it wasn't simply a matter of hearing the beep without the shock and thus learning that it wasn't scary.

So why the difference between these two groups of rats? Could hearing the beep just prior to the anisomycin injection really have had such a big impact on what was remembered?

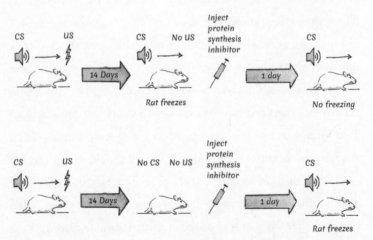

Fig. 25   Reconsolidation of conditioned freezing in rats

Karim Nader and colleagues from McGill University, who conducted this research, think it could. They suggest that hearing
the beep caused the memory to be retrieved (just like getting
that book out of the archives), but when the rat tried to put
it away again, he couldn't because consolidation requires the
construction of new proteins and the anisomycin injection prevented this from happening. Basically, the injection prevented
the book from being reshelved, and therefore the memory got
lost and was forgotten. The group that didn't hear the sound
before the anisomycin injection didn't have this problem because
their memory was never retrieved: It was still safely stored away
in the archive, so the anisomycin had no impact on it at all. It
was this surprising observation—that, once reactivated, memories have to be actively processed if they are to be remembered
later—that led to the concept we call reconsolidation.

In rats at least, memories appear to be somewhat fragile after they've been retrieved. But why is this important, and what
does it mean for humans? It may be that this memory lability
is important because it gives us a chance to change memories,
and sometimes that is essential. We often want to update our
knowledge (imagine a social situation in which two friends were
a couple for three years, but now they have separated and she is
seeing someone else), link previously unrelated concepts together
(she is actually seeing a colleague you knew from a completely
different social circle, so she has become part of that group as
well), and sometimes even remove unwanted components (for
instance, the strongly negative emotion associated with really
horrific memories like the one you formed of the little girl dying
in your arms). It is for the removal of unwanted information that

the reconsolidation concept has proven really useful. This is because it looks as though reconsolidation can be used to selectively wipe out the most negative aspects of really disturbing memories.

As a matter of fact, clinicians have even started using reconsolidation as a treatment for PTSD. Treatments of this type usually rely upon a combination of REM-like eye movements and talking therapy in which the patient imagines the traumatic scene they are trying to get rid of. It isn't entirely clear what the eye movements do in this therapy, but some argue that they help to minimize physiological responses associated with the emotions in the memory. In this way, participants are able to call back a traumatic memory *without* evoking the associated autonomic responses (just as they would have done by replaying it in REM sleep, where norepinephrine levels are low), this means newer consolidation can replace the old memory with a less emotionally charged version. Although the connection between eye movements and reduced physiological response remains somewhat murky (and in fact many people argue that the eye movements are unnecessary), this treatment is surprisingly effective, with just a single session completely curing profound PTSD in some cases. Such results provide convincing evidence that reconsolidation can alter human memories and specifically the traumatic memories which cause problems in PTSD.

What does reconsolidation have to do with sleep? There is actually a strong link here. A study by Matt Walker and his colleagues at Berkeley showed that retrieving memories before sleep can influence the way they are consolidated during subsequent snoozing.[7] Instead of injecting a protein synthesis inhibitor, this study used interference, or learning another memory which is very similar but not quite the same as the original one, as a way of disrupting the initial memory. The paradigm was as follows: On the first day, people learned to tap their fingers in a particular sequence (let's call it sequence A, 4–1–3–2–4, for example, if the fingers on one hand minus the thumb are numbered 1 to 4). People had to tap out this sequence as fast as possible. They were given time to practice this before being tested to see how fast they could do it. You might remember from chapter 1 that if people are allowed to consolidate this type of sequence overnight they get faster at it—up to 20 percent faster, in fact (Fig. 26a). People in this study didn't just learn sequence A; they learned a second sequence as well (let's call it sequence B)—imagine this was 3–1–4–2–1, for instance. The problem here is that, if the sequences were learned one after the other, then the second sequence interfered with the first, such that memory for the first sequence didn't improve overnight. However, if sequence A is learned on day 1 and sequence B is learned on day 2, then on day 3 people show improvement on *both* sequences (Fig. 26b). Here comes the trick (and the link to reconsolidation). If sequence A is learned on day 1 and practiced just once on day 2 right before sequence B is learned, then on day 3 sequence A shows no improvement (Fig. 26c). This might be pretty confusing when you read it, but take a look at the figure to get a better picture.

If you think about it, this is just like the experiments in which anisomycin was injected into the amygdala right after rats were reminded of fearful associations with a sound: The memory for sequence A was (however briefly) called back from the library stacks of the mind, and then, before it could be reshelved,

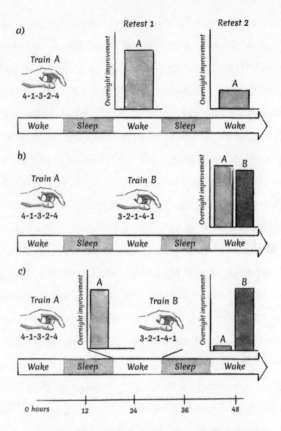

Fig. 26   Reconsolidation in humans, demonstrated
using interference between two tapping sequences

sequence B came along and scrambled it. However, if people were able to sleep between learning sequence A and learning sequence B, there was no interference, suggesting that sleep allowed (or even facilitated) a thorough tidying away of sequence A before sequence B was learned.

The idea that sleep consolidates things such that they aren't so easy to disrupt doesn't just hold up for finger tapping. Another study showed similar findings using the memory task, which we talked about in chapter 6. In this task, eight pairs of identical pictures that resemble playing cards are set out in a 4 × 4 array (so there are 16 cards but only 8 different images). At the start of the game, the cards are all face down so you can only see their backs, which are all identical. The task is to collect pairs by flipping over one card and then trying to remember where its match is and choosing that card next. People who play the game gradually form a representation of where all the pictures are, so they can easily make pairs every time, and they tend to remember this better if they are allowed to sleep in between their initial attempt at the game and a next try in which the cards are laid out in the same pattern as before. This consolidation-related memory advantage can be boosted by triggering replay of memory of the card game in sleep. This can be done by presenting a specific smell (in this case a rose scent) while people play the task initially and then re-presenting that same smell to them while they sleep afterward (see chapter 12 for more on this).[8]

How does this relate to the reactivation of memories? A more recent study used exactly this paradigm but added cognitive interference.[9] Everyone first played the card game with cards set up in array A and with rose scent in the background. Half the participants then slept for 40 minutes, while the other half stayed awake. During these 40 minutes, everybody smelled the rose odor again, which should have triggered reactivation of the memory. Next, everybody did what we call an interference task, something designed to disrupt the memories that had already been formed. They played the game again, but this time the second card in every pair was in a different location; they had to learn a whole new spatial setup, which presumably disrupted their memory for the original layout. After learning the new setup, everybody was tested on the original layout. How did performance differ between people who had slept before the interference task and people who had stayed awake? Both should have reactivated the memory representation of the first spatial layout just before they learned the new layout and thus presumably experienced interference. Fascinatingly, however, people who slept before the interference task did markedly better on the final test than people who remained awake. Just like the finger-tapping study described above, this finding suggests that sleep acts to stabilize the original memory, making it less susceptible to subsequent interference. Reactivation of the memory during that sleep doesn't appear to make it labile in the way that reactivation during wake presumably would. Instead, sleepy reactivation appears to boost the stabilization process.

All in all, the evidence in favor of memory reconsolidation is overpowering. Memories really do become labile, and thus fragile, every single time we use them. Once in this state they can easily be disrupted, either by newer learning which interferes with them or by chemicals that prevent them from being stored (or reshelved). Reconsolidation provides the perfect mechanism for updating memories. Sleep, on the other hand, appears to be critical for "battening down the hatches," or strengthening a memory such that it is more resistant to interference (so long as it doesn't get reactivated in subsequent wake, that is). Critically, reconsolidation also provides the missing mechanism for the overnight therapy concept: Reactivation of memories in sleep without the associated bodily responses essentially disarms the memory, stripping it of emotional content.

CRITICISMS OF THE THEORY

Although overnight therapy is compelling as an idea and fits beautifully with the literature on reconsolidation, there is a fly in the ointment. Quite a few studies have failed to show the expected effects of sleep on emotional intensity ratings and responses in the amygdala. For instance, one study found that people rated images as less emotive after *wake* and observed no change in ratings of emotion across sleep.[10] This finding opposes data showing that emotional images are less jarring after sleep. This negative finding is especially convincing because it supports an older study in which picture ratings taken before and after REM-poor early night sleep revealed that, rather than decreasing, the emotional responses evoked by the pictures increased over this period.[11] Unfortunately, the balance of evidence seems to lean heavily against the idea of overnight therapy. Memories simply do not lose their emotionality after a night of sleep in normal healthy people. In fact, recent research in rats has shown that *depriving* animals of sleep for a few hours after a traumatic experience significantly reduces the probability that the trauma will be remembered later on, suggesting that sleep may actually *strengthen* pernicious memories in some cases.

But what about those tantalizing data described at the start of this chapter, which did show a reduction in emotionality, and in amygdala response, after sleep? These findings are real and certainly shouldn't be overlooked. The fact is, this type of conflict in the scientific literature may be confusing, but it is also exciting—how can we explain such apparently different results?

One answer could relate to memory. In the study that showed reduced emotional reactions after sleep, participants weren't asked to remember anything, and they were not tested on memory. On the other hand, all of the studies that showed increased emotional ratings and amygdala responses after sleep specifically examined memory. In these studies, people were presented with emotional images, or something that had been associated with these images, and asked whether they remembered them. This means people were actively trying to conjure up memories (and very likely mental images) of the pictures they had been shown. Could it be this act of conjuring which leads to the extra emotional response? After all, if people remember an image better after sleep they probably remember how they felt about it better too—but that doesn't necessarily mean they still feel the same way as they did originally, it just means they can recollect those prior feelings more clearly. In fact, you could almost say people who are being tested for memory will be trying to re-create the original scenario, complete with a representation of the feeling that was present the first time around. This could explain why better memory after sleep is also associated with a stronger emotional response.

Another answer could relate to stress.[12] A study by Hein van Marle and colleagues at the Donders Institute for Brain Cognition and Behaviour in the Netherlands showed that the extent to which emotional reactions are toned down across sleep relates directly to stress levels during sleep. This study used pictures in exactly the same way as the studies mentioned above, and participants were aware that they would have a memory test after waking up. However, in half of the people who participated, the stress hormone cortisol was artificially elevated during sleep. Although participants did not rate images for emotional intensity, the elevated cortisol changed the way negative memories were processed in sleep. Amygdala responses were increased during postsleep recognition of negative images in participants who had normal cortisol levels but not in participants with artificially high cortisol. This is a fascinating finding, because it suggests that the way sleep impacts upon emotional representations depends upon how stressed you are while you sleep. This idea fits perfectly with the literature on PTSD, since people who have abnormally low cortisol are much more likely to develop this disorder than people with normal levels of cortisol. None of the other studies discussed in this section measured cortisol levels, so it is difficult to know whether differences in this stress hormone could explain the disparate results. It is possible that participants in the study by Walker and colleagues who showed a decrease in emotional responses after sleep were simply much more stressed than participants in the other studies. After all, this work was conducted in a highly competitive university environment at Berkeley—maybe these participants were students undergoing abnormal amounts of chronic stress.

SUMMING UP

This chapter has introduced "overnight therapy," the idea that sleep disarms dangerous memories, helping us to cope with traumatic or unhappy situations. We looked at memory lability and how the reconsolidation of memories during sleep may allow them to be modified such that emotional content is dampened or removed. We also summarized some of the evidence which contradicts this theory by showing that sleep can in fact *increase* emotional responses to unpleasant pictures seen the day before. Two possible explanations for the conflicting data were discussed—one relates to whether participants were explicitly asked to remember the emotional stimuli they saw before sleep, and the other to stress levels during sleep.

Whatever the reason for the difference in opinions, it is critical that neuroscientists solve this conundrum since the overnight therapy theory suggests that people who have been traumatized should be allowed to sleep so as to dissociate emotion from the traumatic memory while the opposing view suggests that these same trauma victims should be kept awake in order to prevent negative impressions from being strengthened. Which method would you subscribe to after experiencing the traumatic traffic accident and the dying young girl?

eleven

good sleepers and bad sleepers

GOD DIDN'T MAKE US ALL EQUAL.
This is as true of sleep as it is of anything else. Sleep patterns and characteristics vary across different people. You probably know people who only sleep four or five hours a night and others who seem to need ten or more hours of sleep (and no, I don't just mean teenagers—they form their own category; some adults also need this much sleep). You probably also know some of those irritating people who wake up early every morning brimming with energy and the desire to talk to their slower, more grumpy, late-sleeping counterparts who stayed up because they feel best after 2 a.m. These are all superficial differences in sleep patterns and thus easy to identify, but there are also other, more integral, differences that can only be picked up when sleep is properly monitored and analyzed. For instance, some people have higher

sleep efficiency, meaning they spend a greater part of the time between going to bed and getting up in the morning actually sleeping. Others spend ages getting to sleep, wake up frequently during the night and toss and turn, or lie in bed for hours in the morning after they've awakened. Still more intrinsic to sleep, some people have more of those high-frequency oscillations we call sleep spindles, and some people have higher percentages of REM or slow wave sleep. It is impossible to know all of the ways in which these differences influence people, but we do have hints about some of their impacts.

LARKS AND OWLS

The existence of morning people and evening people has probably been common knowledge for as long as humans have lived together in groups. Even though we all sleep and wake according to a cycle of roughly 24 hours, there is always someone who wants to stay up long after the sun has set and "normal" people have gone to bed. These people (colloquially dubbed night owls) often simply feel more alert at night. They may be able to concentrate better, feel they can do their best work then, or simply enjoy being awake more at night than during most parts of the day. Conversely, there are always a few bubbly, energetic morning people around. These "larks" typically bounce out of bed well before the average person would want to open their eyes. Fortunately, natural selection seems to have worked against those larks who tried to awaken people with more normal rhythms too early in the morning. Perhaps for this reason they make up quite a small percentage of the population (just 10 percent).

Seriously, though, people vary in the times they like to sleep and wake—this has been the case throughout history. What's new, however, is the recent discovery that the tendency toward being a lark or an owl is genetically determined in a similar way to the tendency to have blue or green eyes. The gene that governs sleep/wake predisposition is called Period, or PER for short. Like the gene for eye color, it comes in two different types (let's call them PERl, which causes people to have larkish tendencies, and PERo, which causes them to have owlish tendencies). You probably know that we have two copies of all our genes, which means we have two copies of PER as well. The trick, however, is that these copies don't have to be the same: If you have two copies of PERl, you'll be a lark. If you have two copies of PERo, you'll be an owl. But if you have one copy of each (which is what 50 percent of the population has), you'll be somewhere in between. This works for eye color too, by the way: If you have two copies of EYE-COLORg, you'll have green eyes. Two copies of EYE-COLORb you'll have blue eyes, and a copy of each you'll have brown eyes.

The scientists who discovered that sleep-wake tendencies are predicted by the PER gene didn't stop there. They went on to look closely at genetic larks and owls and compare them on all sorts of behavioral tasks. This research revealed lots of differences. First, larks don't just like to get up early; they also get tired much earlier in the day than owls, and they can't handle sleep deprivation—it disrupts their concentration much more than it would for an owl. On the other hand, although owls hate to get up early, and often can't really function in the morning, they handle sleep deprivation very well and can get on with things just fine even when they are deprived (up to a limit, of course).

LIFESPAN CHANGES

Sleep patterns don't just vary from one individual to another; they vary within an individual as they age (Fig. 27). Some of you may be thinking, Well, I *used* to be an owl when I was younger, but now I think I'm more of a lark. That is, you used to love to stay out late or just stay up late at home reading or watching TV and then really struggle to get up in the morning; now you happily succumb to slumber as early as 9 or 10 p.m. and then get out of bed at 5 or 6 a.m. with little difficulty. This isn't surprising at all. Even though circadian types are genetically determined, tendencies vary in a predictable way across the lifetime, especially for the majority of people who are neither true lark nor true owl but actually have a copy of both types of genes (PERl and PERo).

For instance, while babies tend to get huge amounts of sleep (about 16 to 18 hours for a newborn and 14 to 15 hours for a one-year-old), this pattern gradually tails off to the average 7 to 8 hours needed by an adult. Interestingly, adolescents actually need more sleep than slightly younger children, approximately 8.5 to 9.25 hours per night. Adolescents also shift their sleep-wake cycle slightly later than either adults or younger children, typically feeling most alert late in the evening and preferring to wake up and go to bed several hours later than average. This circadian shift has been blamed for the poor performance of teenagers who are forced to arrive at school early in the morning.

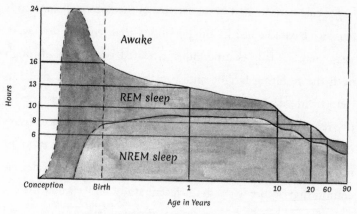

Fig. 27   Lifespan changes in sleep structure

In fact some school systems have experimentally shifted the academic day several hours later and found a dramatic improvement in scores. A good example of this comes from schools in Minnesota, where shifting the morning start from roughly 7:15 a.m. to 8:40 a.m. resulted in improved alertness in class, improved grades, improved attendance, decreased tardiness, reduced visits to the school nurse, and improved overall behavior and atmosphere over a three-year period.

Perhaps the most dramatic change in sleep across the lifespan occurs as we age. This change is associated not only with a gradual reduction in the time spent asleep (from seven to eight hours as a young adult to five to six hours after the age of 60) but also with a specific reduction in slow wave sleep. By age 74, slow wave sleep is often completely absent. It is unclear whether this loss is due to a reduced need for that particular type of sleep, perhaps because of reduced physical activity and learning during the day or results instead from a loss of the ability to sustain such large-scale coordinated brain activity. If the latter explanation is true, we have to consider the possibility that reduced slow wave sleep may actually compound age-related problems—through both the resulting fatigue and also the poor memory that can stem from a lack of consolidation. It is even possible that relative reduction in the amount of slow wave sleep older people get compared to younger people eventually leads to some types of neural damage and might be linked to the gradual neurodegeneration that occurs with age. A recent study showed that the extent of medial prefrontal cortex atrophy in older adults predicted not only reductions in the slow waves they obtained but also a reduction in the amount of consolidation that occurred during that sleep.[1] These are open topics of current research, however, so we will have to wait some time before the true causes and effects of sleep reduction in aging are known.

SPINDLES AND IQ

People differ wildly in the number of sleep spindles they produce. You'll remember that spindles are the fast (12–16 Hz) but low-amplitude oscillations that occur in stage 2 non-REM and occasionally in slow wave sleep. Sleep spindles are never seen in wake or REM sleep. They increase toward the end of the night and (crucially) vary widely across people. However, spindle patterns are so extremely consistent within an individual that they are sometimes referred to as an electrophysiological fingerprint.

Sleep spindles aren't just interesting to us sleep-geeks who love to watch them appear on our computer screens while our hapless victims slumber peacefully—they are interesting to everyone, and here's why. The number of sleep spindles your brain produces predicts IQ scores as well as more general measures of intelligence. This has been examined with a range of tests, and the finding is consistent: Sleep spindle density (that's the number of spindles per unit time) predicts Full-scale IQ and Performance IQ but not Verbal IQ, meaning spindles predict the ability to learn certain types of skilled tasks. The supersmart aren't the only ones who have lots of spindles. People with learning disabilities also score high here, and their spindles have abnormally high amplitudes, earning them the name *extreme spindles*. Just as it's unclear what spindles are doing in those with off-the-charts IQ scores, it is unclear what they are doing in people with learning disabilities, however it seems unlikely that the extra spindles serve the same purpose in these two groups.

Spindle density also increases after learning, but this only seems to happen if the learning was a bit of a challenge, and the increases don't just happen all over the brain: They seem to be limited to structures that were associated with the learned task. For example, if you learn to play a piece on the piano using your left hand, spindles will increase over your right motor cortex (which controls the left side of your body) during your next night of sleep. It even looks as though the extent to which they increase predicts the extent to which your piano playing will improve overnight—in other words, how much better you'll be the next day.

Putting this information about spindles and learning together raises an important question about whether a person's baseline spindle count predicts their ability to consolidate memories across sleep. If we add the known relationship between

spindles and IQ to this mix we may start to wonder whether the
ability to consolidate might predict general intelligence in some
manner—a tantalizing possibility.

INSOMNIA

Arguably, the worst kind of sleep is the kind that leaves you
feeling tired. This type of sleep is typically referred to as nonrestorative sleep and is well known to many of us and is clinically
acknowledged (even though it isn't technically a clinical condition). Nonrestorative sleep seems a bit enigmatic at first—people
with this problem don't have any trouble falling asleep, staying
asleep, or generally getting enough sleep—but they just don't
feel rested when they wake up. When closely examined, people
with frequent nonrestorative sleep turned out to have the same
types of problems as people with insomnia, e.g., feeling sleepy,
tired, or low energy during the day; having poor concentration
or memory, or needing more effort to get things done; and feeling irritable, stressed, and moody. So why isn't sleep working its
normal magic for these people? We don't have a complete answer
to this question yet, but at least part of the problem is thought
to be in the slow waves. Even though nonrestorative sleepers are
technically *sleeping* for the same amount of time as everyone else,
there is growing evidence that they aren't getting the normal dose
of slow wave sleep. Most examinations of this idea have looked
at nonrestorative sleep in insomniacs. (Insomnia is defined as
the *perception* that you're not getting enough sleep, even if you
technically are, so while some insomniacs truly don't sleep, or
at least have serious problems falling asleep and staying asleep,

others feel tired despite sleeping—i.e., they have nonrestorative sleep.) These nonrestorative insomniacs typically show less slow wavelike brain activity and more wakelike brain activity during sleep. You could almost say they aren't fully asleep. Since slow waves serve a critical role in resetting the brain so that it is refreshed and ready for a new day of learning, it isn't surprising that missing out on these waves might leave people feeling tired, out of sorts, and unable to concentrate. The idea that slow waves are responsible for these problems is supported by the observation that using drugs to increase this type of brain activity goes a long way toward reversing these symptoms.

OTHER SLEEP DISORDERS

Of course, more serious sleep disorders can lead to sleep with even worse consequences than being tired. For instance, people with sleep-related eating disorders regularly get out of bed in their sleep and help themselves to the contents of their fridge or cupboard. They usually don't realize this is happening and can grow obese as a result (not to mention the obvious squabbles with partners, family, and flatmates about who ate the chocolate-chip ice cream). Once officially diagnosed, such nocturnal eaters are often instructed to put a padlock on their fridge as the only way of preventing this behavior.

Sleep-related eating disorder is just one manifestation of sleepwalking—or somnambulism—which occurs during the deepest phases of slow wave sleep. Although eating in your sleep can cause problems, it isn't the worst thing that can happen. People can perform even more complex behaviors: For instance, one man went outside, drove more than 30 miles to his in-law's house, and then murdered them with a kitchen knife. This isn't an isolated case—see table 1 for a list of similar incidents and the court verdicts.

SUMMING UP

Clearly people vary hugely in the way they sleep. Some of this variance is due to genetics, but lots of other factors come into play. Age, sex, daily habits, and diet all play a role. Whatever your sleeping style is, remember that it has a big impact on how you interact with the world, from moodiness to memory to the possibility of violent crimes (or glutinous eating) while you snooze. Bearing all of this in mind, perhaps it is worth thinking of ways to improve your sleep—and that is the topic of chapters 12 and 13.

TABLE OF SLEEP CRIMES

Violent Behavior	Circumstances	Evaluation	Verdict of Court
Shot hotel porter 3 times	Porter entered darkened hotel room unannounced and attempted to awaken defendant	Provoked by porter	Convicted and reversed on appeal
Assaulted 2 police officers	Police officers found intoxicated defendant asleep in car, attempted to wake up	Provoked by police officers	Not reported
Shot girlfriend	Disturbed by noise while asleep, jumped up with gun and started firing. Found girlfriend dead on bed	Provoked by noise?	Acquitted
Beat victim with fists; stabbed to death with knife	Victim attempted to arouse defendant from sleep	Provoked by victim	Convicted and reversed on appeal
Stabbed husband 3 times, back, chest, thigh	Suffering from cough, shared bed with husband. Awakened by cough? Where did knife come from?	Possibly provoked by cough	Not reported
Knight stabbed friend to death	Was asleep when friend tried to awaken him	Provoked	Not reported
Killed wife with axe	Defendant was awakened by noise around midnight. Grabbed axe and attacked "stranger" in room	Provoked	Not reported

(continues)

TABLE OF SLEEP CRIMES (CONTINUED)

Violent Behavior	Circumstances	Evaluation	Verdict of Court
Strangled prostitute while intoxicated	Awakened to find hands around neck of woman he had slept with. Involvement of alcohol	Provoked??	Acquitted
Killed employee entering office with gun	Night shift supervisor fell asleep in office. Approximately 30 minutes later, employee entered office and awakened him. Pulled gun in confusion and fired	Provoked	Not reported
Stabbed to death	Boy shared room with defendant along with 13 others. He tried to pick up something next to the sleeping defendant. Defendant was aroused by disturbance and grabbed knife and stabbed him	Provoked	Not reported

M. R. Pressman, "Disorders of Arousal From Sleep and Violent Behavior: The Role of Physical Contact and Proximity," *Sleep* 30, 8 (August 1, 2007): 1039–1047.

twelve

getting the most out
of your sleep

SOMETIMES YOU MAY WANT YOUR sleep to serve a very specific function. Maybe you've had a fight with your partner and could really use some REM sleep to help you deal with the difficult emotions, or maybe you're studying for an exam and would love a load of slow wave sleep to strengthen up your newly learned memories. Is there some way to make sure you get the right kind of sleep? And is there a way to ensure it is the memories you want strengthened, not the memories you consider unimportant or even destructive, which get replayed while you slumber? The short answer is yes—well, maybe. The long answer is below.

TIMES TO SLEEP

Once you understand its role in memory consolidation, sleep can almost be thought of as a type of medication, e.g., "Take this much slow wave sleep in order to achieve that result." Of course this quickly gets complicated because your brain is essentially freewheeling when you sleep. How do you tell it, "I want more REM and less sleep spindles, please!"?

One good trick is in the timing. Sleep stages are so tightly linked to our 24-hour body clock that napping at different times of day leads to different types of sleep. Napping in the morning will mean you drop into REM, while napping late in the afternoon usually results in slow wave sleep. This is because the sleep need, or physical drive for the different types of sleep, varies across the day. During the night we've normally had a good six to eight hours of snoozing, including all the slow wave sleep our brains could possibly want. By the morning, when our 90-minute cycle of the four sleep stages restarts for the fourth or fifth time, we're likely to skip this deep sleep stage and go straight to REM instead. This is the reason why people get so much REM in the second part of the night. They are out of slow wave sleep mode and in REM mode. It is also the reason why those long lie-ins on the weekend often result in such vivid dreams.

An afternoon nap, on the other hand, is a different kettle of fish. By that time of day you've probably been awake and active for hours, and your brain has built up a genuine *need* for slow wave sleep, so you are likely to plunge into slow wave mode after just a little time in non-REM stages 1 and 2. Where does this need come from? You may remember the synaptic homeostasis model (chapter 5), which proposes that the brain's drive to get slow wave sleep is rooted entirely in the need to downscale synaptic connections that were strengthened through wakeful activities. Whether or not this is true, it is absolutely clear that you will be more likely to enter slow wave sleep and to stay in it for longer late in the day than you will early in the morning.

The really exciting thing about the connection between sleep and your state of mind is that you can manipulate different types of sleep to your advantage. If you want slow wave sleep to strengthen your neural representations of specific bits of knowledge, then it would be sensible to take a nap in the afternoon. On the other hand, if you want to strengthen emotional memories, it might be better to sleep longer in the morning, or take a morning nap. This isn't a hard and fast prescription, of course, but that is because we are still exploring the roles of these various types of sleep. The association between time of day and sleep type is absolutely firm.

TIMES TO LEARN

If you are strategic enough about your memory to be napping at the right time of day to ensure you get the best possible sleep to consolidate a new memory, you will probably also want to optimize the way you learn the specific bits of information which you are trying to target. Newly learned memories are more likely to be replayed when you sleep, so studying immediately before the nap, or at least rehearsing what you've learned before you snooze, is a good idea. This should help to ensure the target knowledge is kept in mind and gets replayed once you are asleep, but it should also ensure that the memories you want to strengthen haven't already been degraded so much by the influx of interfering information that it can't consolidate when you do get to sleep.

This is all very well if you're going to be napping, but things get trickier if you want to strengthen particular memories during overnight sleep. That's because you're likely to be tired in the evening, and being tired makes it harder to learn; even though studying right before you go to bed optimizes consolidation, this type of schedule could also be counterproductive because your brain is less able to code new information in the first place.

FAKING IT (OTHERWISE KNOWN AS ARTIFICIAL SLEEP)

Prior chapters (5, 7, and 8) explained that the huge brain waves found during slow wave sleep are important for consolidation. These waves are created when large populations of neurons fire at the same time. Because neural firing is triggered by a change in the electrical potential across the external membrane of a nerve cell, Lisa Marshall and her colleagues in Lübeck, Germany, decided to see whether they could trigger slow waves artificially by applying carefully timed electrical stimulation to the scalp.[1] To do this, they put large, spongy electrodes on either side of the forehead and injected current through them in pulses that matched the frequency of the large-amplitude oscillations in slow wave sleep (approximately 0.75 Hz). The experiment was a raging success and showed that it is possible to "entrain" slow waves by judiciously injecting current into the brain in this manner (Fig. 28). There were also additional findings: Not only did

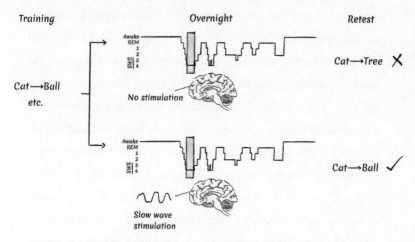

Fig. 28   *Electrical stimulation enhances SWS and memory consolidation*

this current application increase the amount of slow wave sleep people obtained, it also led to superior memory consolidation. Participants were asked to learn a series of word pairs before the experiment (like cat-ball), and their memory was tested the next day. People who had been exposed to the 0.75 Hz stimulation during sleep remembered markedly more than people who had not, suggesting that even these artificial slow waves provide an important benefit for memory.

It may be a relief for some of you to hear that more recent work has outdone the electrical stimulation study by producing very similar results in a much less scary way.[2] Mathias Mölle and colleagues at the University of Tübingen in Germany played very brief tones at a frequency just a little slower than one per second and found that this led to longer and more rhythmic trains of slow waves with higher amplitudes and also to superior memory consolidation.

The idea of triggering a deep sleep and targeted memory consolidation through artificial stimulation conjures up images from science fiction—sleep pods or booths in which people might obtain an artificially stimulated 20-minute snooze for the price of a cup of coffee. Just imagine how popular these would be with overtired office workers, as well as with teachers and librarians who might hope to boost their students' memories through this type of strategic napping. With a bit more development it might also be possible to trigger REM sleep, sleep spindles, and other aspects of sleep—such that electrical stimulation will make the time-based methods for controlling sleep by napping at different times of day look completely old-fashioned. These techniques could be especially important for insomniacs since simple application of electrical current might be able to push them almost immediately into a deep and refreshing synthetic sleep. People with other sleep-related disorders could also benefit markedly; for instance, the correct type of electrical stimulation might prevent people with depression from overconsolidating negative memories during REM sleep and could thus help them to break out of their downward spiral. The science of sleep manipulation has a long way to go, but let's hope this is a true vision of the future.

TRIGGERING MEMORY REPLAY DURING SLEEP

Increasing slow waves by sleeping at the right time and rehearsing your studies immediately before you sleep aren't the only things we can do to improve consolidation while you snooze. You've probably heard the old wives' tale that putting a book under your pillow or playing a tape of what you've learned while you sleep will help you retain this information in the long term. These ideas were poo-pooed by the scientific community for years, but a growing understanding of how memory replay during sleep can strengthen representations is forcing a change in that attitude.

It turns out that memory replay really *can* be intentionally triggered during sleep, and such triggering leads to strengthening of memory representations in the brain. The triggering of memory replay is typically accomplished by re-exposing the sleeper to something that was linked with the target memory (e.g., the memory you want to strengthen). Smells are especially useful for this because they are easily processed by the sleeping brain but are unlikely to wake anyone up. Björn Rasch and his colleagues in Lübeck used the smell of roses to trigger memory replay by simply arranging for this odor to be present in the background while people learned their target task.[3] The task was very similar to the old board game Memory, in which a number of card pairs are laid out, face down, and you have to remember where the second half of each pair is, just by trial and error (Fig. 29). (See chapter 10 for a detailed description.) They then slept for a full night in the lab, and different groups of people were re-exposed to the rose scent at different stages of sleep or wake. The rose smell elicited the recall of the location of the cards in a completely subconscious way without the individuals being aware of it. The next morning everyone was tested on their ability to remember where the card pairs were. People who had smelled roses during slow wave sleep were significantly better at this task than anyone else. This somewhat astounding result was the first indication that there might actually be something in that old wives' tale about sleeping with a book under your pillow or listening to a recording of your lesson. It also raised a lot of questions. What is happening in the brain when people smell this scent during sleep? Does it literally reopen the memory of studying the cards since the two were uploaded into the brain together? Can we see any physical evidence that the rose smell triggers the brain to reactivate the process of studying the cards, and therefore through replay helps consolidate the memory so in the morning you perform better than a rival who wasn't exposed to the rose fragrance during the night? And if so, does this replay somehow predict the memory benefit we see the next day?

A subsequent experiment tried to tackle these questions. People were again asked to play the Memory game while smelling a rose scent, and they were again re-exposed to that scent during slow wave sleep that evening, but this time they were sleeping in a brain scanner. The scanner monitored brain activity both while they smelled the roses and while they didn't. This showed that the hippocampus, which you'll remember is critical

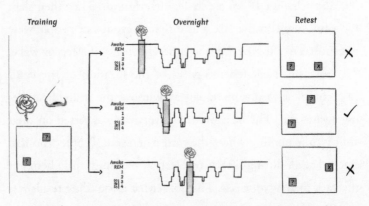

Fig. 29   Using odor to trigger memory reactivation in slow wave sleep

for memory, and especially for spatial memory, was strongly active whenever the rose smell was present in slow wave sleep, suggesting that the smell triggered some form of memory replay. An earlier study had already shown that the extent of hippocampal activity during the slow wave sleep people obtained right after learning to navigate around a virtual town in a 3D video game predicted how much better they got at getting from A to B within that town across a night of sleep.[4] Although the rose scent study didn't show a similar correlation between improvement and replay, it did suggest that the scent triggered the replay, which allowed the memories to be strengthened.

Unfortunately, if you're thinking of trying this trick the next time you study for an exam, I'm afraid you may be disappointed. It turns out that our noses, together with the bits of the brain that process smell, known collectively as the olfactory system, very quickly get used to odors that hang around in the air, so these lose their impact on us almost immediately. Just think of how fast you stop noticing the smell of a strong air freshener in one room of your house if you stay in there for a while. However, if you leave the room, stay away for some time, and then re-enter, the smell hits you again. The organizers of this study took this effect into consideration and figured out a way to keep the scent poignant. They made sure the rose smell didn't lose its impact by using a special device called an olfactometer, which doled out the scent in brief spurts of about 20 seconds, followed by a 20-second break in which the olfactory receptors could reset themselves. Of course, you can buy air fresheners that have timers and release scents at intervals, but it would be difficult to achieve the precision of a laboratory setting at home.

Like smells, sounds have been used to trigger memory replay during sleep, though these obviously have to be played
very softly so as not to create a disturbance that wakes people
up. Sounds are especially good for these kinds of experiments
because it is easy to get participants to learn a whole series of
different things (e.g., a list of words) in which different sounds
are associated with each item. Later on, by replaying some of
the sounds but not others, experimenters can strategically trigger reactivation of just *some* of the memories that were learned,
or even different subsets of these memories, in different stages of
sleep and then look at how this triggering predicts recollection
the next day. This is a really valuable strategy because it quickly
shows whether the triggering really works.

In one famous study using this approach, participants saw
a set of pictures, each of which was placed in a very specific
location on the computer screen, and each of which was paired
with a related sound (the picture of a kitten was paired with
a meow, the picture of a kettle with a whistle, etc.).[5] Half of
the sounds were then replayed softly through speakers while the
volunteers were deep in slow wave sleep. When tested the next
day, sure enough, people were better at putting the objects for
which sounds had been replayed in the right screen locations.
This finding was all the more dramatic because the sleep in question was actually a brief 90-minute nap, and the sounds were
only replayed once each. Who would have thought such a small
amount of consolidation could have such a significant impact!

The study of how sound triggers the brain to replay a particular memory has led to a flurry of excitement among those of
us who are searching for ways to improve memory. It sounds so

simple—cram for your Spanish vocabulary test with Mozart in the background and then play the music softly while you sleep to make sure you get 100 percent! A recent follow-up shows that the same principle works for a different type of memory called skill learning—that's the memory we use for riding a bicycle or playing a musical instrument, and also for the finger-tapping task discussed in chapter 1. These skills don't rely upon the same neural mechanisms as the card location game Memory. Skill learning doesn't usually require spatial navigation; instead of involving conscious thought, it is associated with habit or doing things by rote. Instead of the hippocampus, such skills typically draw on an evolutionarily older structure called the basal ganglia. Because they are situated in different parts of the brain, the two types of memory differ in many characteristics. To determine whether procedural memories can be strengthened by triggered replay during sleep, Ken Paller and colleagues from Northwestern University in Chicago used something along the lines of the computer game *Guitar Hero*. In this game, players use a remote control which is likened to a guitar. Each finger is on a button which represents a different string, and players have to play a song by pressing each note at the right time (and holding the button down for the right amount of time too). Because most people probably wouldn't be able to do this very well without some kind of help, there is also a visual display to tell them when to press the buttons and gives them a kind of warning of how soon each press will be. Fascinatingly, if people hear the musical notes from this game during slow wave sleep, they can play the tunes much more accurately the next day.[6] This finding provides conclusive evidence that it isn't just memory for specific events (like the card game) which can be strengthened by triggered re-play during sleep; procedural skill learning is also influenced by this type of treatment. The result may not seem terribly impor-tant at first, but if you think of the implications for athletes who have to learn lots of complex physical skills to do well in their sports, musicians who constantly learn new pieces of music, and even people learning everyday things like how to drive a car, then you may begin to understand why a simple method for improved learning in all these cases could be important.

Work in rats has taken an even bigger step toward answering the question of what happens when we try to trigger memory replay with sounds. This work allows us to take a closer look at what individual neurons in the brain are doing during replay since we can stick electrodes into the rat brain without as many ethical qualms as we would have with the human brain. Record-ings from these electrodes have shown that, when played during sleep, sounds which would normally instruct the rat to run to a particular location in space trigger activity in the place cells linked to that particular area.[7] You'll remember from chapter 6 that place cells are very specialized neurons within the hippo-campus that are used in navigation and spatial memory. As a rat moves through space, each place cell will become associated with a specific location and will thereafter only fire when the rat is once again physically present in that place. The fact that playing a sound which was associated with a specific place triggers firing in the appropriate place cells very strongly supports the idea that such sounds trigger a neural-level replay of events. Of course we can't ask the rats if this replay is linked to any form of dreaming, but that would be an obvious next question.

LEARNING IN YOUR SLEEP?

It even looks as though initial learning can happen in our sleep. Anat Arzi and colleagues from the Weizmann Institute of Science in Rehovot, Israel, recently exposed people to pleasant or repugnant odors when they were either awake or asleep.[8] Each odor coincided with a particular sound, such that (if awake) people would easily have learned that one sound means a nice smell while another means a nasty one. People naturally take shallower breaths through their noses (sniffs) when they smell something foul, so this arrangement meant people tended to take shallower sniffs if they heard the sound associated with the foul smell even when that smell wasn't presented. The really important thing was, however, that people did this *even if they were asleep when the sounds and smells were presented.* Excitingly, the association persisted the next day if previously slumbering participants were again made to listen to the offensive sounds. To give an example, someone in the experiment might have been exposed to the foul smell of rotten eggs while a C chord was played on the piano. The rotten egg smell caused them to take shallower sniffs even in their sleep; the next day when they heard the C chord, they also took shallower sniffs without knowing why. In fact, when asked about this, they had no memory whatsoever of hearing sounds in their sleep or for that matter of smelling anything. This means they definitely didn't wake up and learn that way—instead, they formed the association between smell and sound while completely unconscious. This is a really critical finding because it is the first demonstration that new learning (as compared to consolidation) *can* occur during sleep and suggests that sleep could potentially be used to teach people.

SUMMING UP

This chapter has described a handful of ways in which you can manipulate your sleep to facilitate memory. These include simply sleeping at the right time of day, or at the right time with respect to learning, as well as methods for triggering memory replay and slow waves. In fact, there is no reason why we can't combine these ideas and try artificially triggering memory replay at the same time as triggering slow waves. This would provide a sort of double-whammy for memory strengthening. Scientists haven't attempted this yet, but it is an obvious next step, and certainly in the cards.

thirteen

brief notes on how to get the sleep you need

WHAT IF YOU JUST CAN'T SLEEP OR don't sleep enough? It is clear that sleep is absolutely critical to feeling good and being able to function normally. It helps to keep your body healthy by regulating immune function and temperature, and it is also essential for maintaining mood, constructing memories, updating your general world knowledge, and helping you to take an overview of difficult problems. Sleep is sometimes referred to as the best cognitive enhancer on the market—meaning it beats all the drugs hands down. It may even be the key to superior IQ. The bottom line is, sleep is good for you. It is something your body needs and your brain thrives on. None of us can afford to skimp on sleep, but unfortunately in today's stressful 24-hour society, many of us do. This could be due to lack of time, excess stress, or simply a lack of understanding about how to obtain a good night's sleep. There are many simple tricks to improve your sleep. Some are obvious, and some are less well known. Things like room temperature, the food you've eaten, the sounds, light, and smells in your bedroom, and how you tend to use that room can make a huge difference. This final chapter is a sort of guerrilla guide to good practice for sleeping. Many of these ideas will seem like common sense, but if even a few of them are new to you, it might be worth your while to take a quick look.

PSYCHOLOGY

One of the biggest influences on how you sleep is how you actually *feel* about your bed and bedroom. These should be comfortable, not too brightly lit, and strongly associated with sleep. Sliding into a cozy bed in which you only ever sleep (and maybe make love) sends all the right signals to your brain when it is time to switch off. Getting into a bed which you often use for TV watching, working on your laptop, listening to the radio, and/or reading doesn't send the same message. Instead, this kind of multipurpose bed may cause you to feel more awake when you snuggle under the covers, and it could even prevent you from getting a good snooze.

TEMPERATURE

As a rule of thumb, 16 to 19 degrees Celsius (61 to 66 degrees Fahrenheit) is an optimal room temperature for sleep. Your body temperature always cools slightly when you go to sleep, and artificially triggering this cooling can help you to fall asleep because it tricks your body into the right general state for snoozing. A counterintuitive strategy for getting your body to cool down at just the right time is to heat yourself up a little before going to bed. A hot bath starting about an hour and a half before bedtime is one of the best ways to ensure you'll fall asleep. Warming up in the bath means cooling down is more dramatic and effective after you get out (of course, if you don't have a bath you can take a shower instead, and it will heat you up almost as well—but it probably won't be as enjoyable and relaxing!). If neither shower nor bath is available, then a comfortably hot foot bath right before going to bed may also help, as it will dilate the big blood vessels in the feet, which allows your body temperature to cool more effectively once you get into bed.[1]

Subtle heating of the skin on the body trunk (tummy and chest) can also make people fall asleep faster.[2] Making yourself a warm water bottle or soft toy (about 37 degrees Celsius/99 degrees Fahrenheit) and holding it near your belly when you go to bed might help with this. Only do this if it is comfortable though; anything you find uncomfortable is more likely to keep you awake than help you sleep!

LIGHT

Light resets our 24-hour circadian clock and helps to determine when we sleep and wake. A 24-hour circadian cycle, which is strongly controlled by signals from nature such as sunshine and nocturnal darkness, will help you to feel very alert in the daytime and very sleepy at night. You can promote such a cycle by catching some rays of bright blue light (that's the kind of light you get from being outdoors in bright weather, even if it's not especially sunny) during the day,[3] and also making sure you *are not* exposed to this type of light in the evening or during the night. Blue light at night will reset your circadian clock and can wake you up. Unfortunately, both televisions and computers give off blue light. They also stimulate the mind, which doesn't help much when you're trying to switch off. You really shouldn't be using these devices for the last three hours before you sleep. If you insist on using a smart phone or computer, then the screen should be covered with an orange filter, or you could install software which adjusts the screen to cut down blue light (Google this and you'll find several options). If it is impossible for you to turn off all of the blue light which you might encounter in the evening (e.g., your children are watching television, there is a strong light which shines through your windows, or your spouse insists on having a laptop in bed), then you might also consider wearing orange-filtered glasses during the two to three hours immediately prior to bedtime. Wearing these filters has been shown to improve sleep quality and mood,[4] but be aware that it also leads to poorer sleep on the first night or two of use, so some persistence is required.

Your bedroom should be pitch-black during the night. You may want to fit blackout blinds, and if you do so, make sure they don't allow light to creep in around the edges. All lights from electrical appliances should be removed or covered. If you are uncomfortable with total darkness or need to get up during the night, it is best to use a very dim red/orange light which can be switched on from your bed. Light helps us to wake up in the morning, and it is difficult to get out of bed in total darkness. Very dim red/orange lights which gradually come on, starting about half an hour before the alarm goes off, can make it easier to wake up. Luminance can increase more rapidly after the alarm goes off, and blue components can be introduced into the light. If you can arrange for your blinds and curtains to gradually open after your alarm rings and allow natural light to enter this will help you to feel more alert. Half an hour after the alarm sounds the room and bathroom should both be bathed in strong light. This will also help to keep your circadian clock in order. If possible, it is best to make sure you are exposed to bright blue light for at least 30 minutes every morning. Being outside in the sunshine (for example, while you walk to work) would be ideal. Otherwise, consider getting yourself a blue spectrum sun lamp.

SOUND

Loud, sudden, or unpleasant sounds can prevent you from falling asleep, alter the structure of your sleep, and even wake you up. Because it is difficult to achieve total silence, many sleep experts recommend the usage of a constant, low-intensity masking sound such as pink or white noise (both of which sound more or less like a radio tuned in between stations) to dull the impact of any external sounds. There is evidence that constant white noise successfully masks out background sounds that might otherwise be disturbing[5] and other evidence that pink noise makes it easier to fall asleep.[6]

Some people claim that specially designed audio tracks can also be used to entrain brain activity into the right frequency for sleep. Such ideas have led to the installation of beautiful soundscapes involving birdsong, waves, and even snoring in a few UK hospitals. The link between these kinds of sounds and the auditory tones that have recently been shown to amplify slow waves (see chapter 12) has yet to be explored, but if you have trouble falling asleep you could certainly consider listening to soothing audio tracks of this type—or even the binaural beats "deep sleep" tracks which are heavily advertised on the Internet.

SMELL

It is very important that your bedroom feels fresh, with plenty of clean air. Avoid stuffiness or overuse of perfumes or air fresheners. Many claims have been made about the soporific power of scents such as jasmine, lavender, and valerian. There is scant evidence to support them; a few studies have suggested that a faint scent of valerian can be helpful in the promotion of snoozing, but there is little or no data showing that other odors have the same effect.[7] Before you get too disheartened about this, it is worth mentioning that administering pleasant smells during sleep does lead to more pleasant dreams.[8] If you want to test this out and see if it improves your nocturnal experience you could get an air freshener to switch on about halfway through the night, as the majority of dreams occur after this point. Because we become accustomed to odors very quickly, this will be much more likely to work if you can program your air freshener so that it switches off and on every few minutes. Although the scent of roses is the only one that has been specifically linked to pleasant dreams, there's no reason to think this wouldn't be true for all appealing smells—so why not experiment and settle on whatever (if anything) works for you? Smells of lemon or peppermint can improve your mood while waking and getting up, so you could also consider switching to one of these scents when the alarm goes off.

FOOD

What you eat in the three to five hours leading up to bedtime has a strong impact on how well you will sleep. This is because foods contain chemicals and proteins that can either promote or interfere with your sleep. A medium-size meal of sleep-inducing foods eaten four to five hours before bedtime followed by a small snack about an hour before lights-out is probably the best recipe for a good night of sleep. Sleep-promoting foods include chamomile tea, warm milk, cottage cheese, soy milk, plain yogurt, honey, turkey, tuna fish, bananas, potatoes, oatmeal, almonds, flaxseeds, sunflower seeds, whole-wheat bread, peanut butter, low-fat cheese, and tofu. For dinner, a meal that is high in complex carbohydrates and has a small amount of protein would be ideal.

This really goes without saying, but for the sake of completeness, I should also mention that there are plenty of foods that will keep you awake or at least lead to disrupted sleep. These foods include coffee (or anything with caffeine, including chocolate—sorry!) and alcohol. Foods with the amino acid tyramine, which inhibits sleep, are also on the naughty list. These include peppers, smoked meats, and fish.

Finally, as many of you may have found from unpleasant past experiences, a very heavy meal less than three hours prior to bed can also keep you awake. This is because digestive activity can leave you feeling uncomfortably full or, even worse, cause heartburn. Eating fatty or spicy foods is particularly likely to lead to problems.

TIMING AND NAPPING

As discussed in chapter 11, humans have been programmed genetically to require a set amount of sleep per day. Some of us are long sleepers and some short. Some (larks) function better in the morning than at night while others (owls) have the opposite preference. While these tendencies can be adapted during our lifetime, the basic patterns are embedded in our genetic structure. The timing of our sleep is regulated by light, but this influence decreases as we age. This accounts for a less regular sleep pattern in the elderly and those with some forms of visual impairment since they may not be able to process light in the normal way.

We are programmed to be diurnal. That is, we sleep in the night and wake in the day. Our natural pattern is 8 hours sleep and 16 hours wake, but modern society has stolen some of this sleep, and many people have become adapted to 7 hours sleep and 17 hours wake. If you allow yourself to take some of this sleep in the afternoon (as a Mediterranean nap) or evening (TV nap), you will have a reduced drive for deep sleep during the night. This may result in a broken night and a general frustration that you cannot get to sleep easily or that you are waking too early in the morning. The converse is also true. If you go to bed too early and get up too late you probably won't sleep especially well. This could show up as either taking a long time to drop off to sleep or frequent arousals, both of which would be classified as insomnia. Paradoxically, reducing the time spent in bed can increase the quality of sleep in such cases and may therefore help reduce daytime tiredness.

The solution to this type of insomnia may be to try to avoid daytime napping and reduce time in bed to less than seven hours by retiring later than usual. It is also essential to get out of bed at the standard time and avoid napping the following day. If you manage this for several days, with no more than five or six hours of sleep opportunity, you may be able to reward yourself by retiring 15 minutes earlier for one week. Repeating this exercise several times over a month or more will allow you to determine the minimum amount of time you need for sleep with early sleep onset and unbroken sleep, which in turn may improve the overall quality of the sleep you experience.

INTRUSIVE THOUGHTS AND RUMINATING MINDS

It is difficult to fall asleep if your mind is whirring away at a hundred miles per hour. If you try to sleep at the wrong time or simply go to bed when you're not tired, then you may find your brain is unhelpfully active. If people are not sufficiently sleepy when they get into bed their minds tend to become active and to develop ruminating thoughts: "Why can't I sleep—I need sleep but cannot get it—if I cannot sleep I will not be able to function tomorrow, I need sleep to be able to take my exam tomorrow," etc., etc., etc. The longer you allow these thoughts to remain, the more difficult it will be to get to sleep. If these thoughts persist for more than 30 minutes, then you should consider getting up and (while keeping warm, obviously!) doing a relaxing activity which may help you to dispel some of the ruminations: Read a book or plan for tomorrow until you feel relaxed and sleepy (no tea, coffee, or alcohol please!) and then go back to bed. If you do this you must still arise at the usual morning time and avoid taking any naps to compensate for the missed sleep.

Short-term insomnia, though upsetting and inconvenient, is not a real problem. Habitual long-term insomnia, on the other hand, needs attention.

SNORING AND SLEEP APNEA

If you snore loudly, often need to go to the toilet at night, or commonly wake with a morning headache and a dry mouth and feel tired during the day, you may be suffering from sleep-disordered breathing. Some of these symptoms can be relieved by aggressive weight loss programs, but in many instances, it would be prudent to have them checked out by your doctor or request a referral to a sleep clinic.

SUMMING UP

This book has described some of the intricacies, fascinations, and mysteries of sleep. We have talked about the ubiquity of sleep in the animal kingdom, as well as impacts of sleep deprivation on mind and body. We have looked at the complex and highly structured series of neural states that our brain passes through during sleep, as well as examining the brain systems which turn sleep on and off. We have looked at the ways in which sleep benefits memory, as well as the way it may act in construction of semantic knowledge, insight, and creativity. We have looked at the neural basis of dreaming, and how dreams relate to memories and memory consolidation. We have also considered the ways in which sleep interacts with emotions—controlling our moods and influencing how we feel about traumatic experiences. We have considered the differences in people's individual sleep patterns and thought about how this may impact upon their minds, memories, and mentalities. Finally, we've looked at ways to enhance sleep and thus harness some of its benefits in a calculated fashion. If nothing else, this book should have convinced you that sleep is essential to our physical and mental well-being. You may never use artificial techniques to trigger memory replay or slow oscillations while you sleep, but I hope you will at least consider giving sleep some kind of priority in your life. The tips in this last chapter—our guerrilla guide to getting sleep—should help to ensure you can do this if desired.

notes

CHAPTER 1: WHY SLEEP?

1. J. Horne, "Petunias, One-Eyed Ducks, and Roly-Poly Mice," *Sleepfaring* (Oxford: Oxford University Press, 2006), 1–15.
2. A. A. Borberley and J. L. Valatx, "Sleep in Marine Mammals," *Sleep Mechanisms* (Munich: Springer, 1984), 227.
3. Quoted in Matthew P. Walker, "The Role of Sleep in Cognition and Emotion," The Year in Cognitive Neuroscience 2009: *Ann. N.Y. Acad. Sci.* 1156: 168–197 (2009).
4. John G. McCoy and Robert E. Strecker, "The Cognitive Cost of Sleep Lost," *Neurobiology of Learning and Memory* 96 (2011): 564–582.
5. A. Rechtschaffen, B. M. Bergmann, C. A. Everson, C. A. Kushida, and M. A. Gilliland, "Sleep Deprivation in the Rat: X. Integration and Discussion of the Findings," *Sleep* 12, no. 1 (2002): 68–87.
6. G. Gulevich, W. Dement, and L. Johnson, "Psychiatric and EEG Observations on a Case of Prolonged (264 hours) Wakefulness," *Arch. Gen. Psychiatry* 15 (1966): 29–35.
7. M. P. Walker and R. Stickgold, "It's Practice, With Sleep, That Makes Perfect: Implications of Sleep-Dependent Learning and Plasticity for Skill Performance," *Clin. Sports Med.* 24, ix (2005): 301–317.

CHAPTER 2: HOW DO WE KNOW SLEEP IS IMPORTANT FOR THE BRAIN?

1. W. D. Killgore, "Effects of Sleep Deprivation on Cognition," *Prog. Brain Res.* 185 (2010): 105–129.
2. Ibid.

3. S. S. Yoo, P. T. Hu, N. Gujar, F. A. Jolesz, and M. P. Walker, "A Deficit in the Ability to Form New Human Memories Without Sleep," *Nat. Neurosci.* 10 (2007): 385–392.
4. M. P. Walker, "The Role of Sleep in Cognition and Emotion," *Ann. N. Y. Acad. Sci.* 1156 (2009): 168–197.

CHAPTER 4: HOW THE BRAIN CONTROLS SLEEP

1. K. O. Newman, *Encephalitis Lethargica, Sequelae and Treatment* (trans.) (London: Oxford University Press, 1931).

CHAPTER 5: MENTAL SPRING CLEANING WHILE YOU SLEEP

1. G. Tononi and C. Cirelli, "Sleep and Synaptic Homeostasis: A Hypothesis," *Brain Res. Bull.* 62 (2003): 143–150.
2. D. Bushey, G. Tononi, and C. Cirelli, "Sleep and Synaptic Homeostasis: Structural Evidence in *Drosophila*," *Science* 332 (2011): 1576–1581.
3. R. Huber, M. F. Ghilardi, M. Massimini, and G. Tononi, "Local Sleep and Learning," *Nature* 430 (2004): 78–81.
4. R. Huber et al., "Arm Immobilization Causes Cortical Plastic Changes and Locally Decreases Sleep Slow Wave Activity," *Nat. Neurosci.* 9 (2006): 1169–1176.
5. R. Huber et al., "Measures of Cortical Plasticity after Transcranial Paired Associative Stimulation Predict Changes in Electroencephalogram Slow-wave Activity during Subsequent Sleep," *J. Neurosci.* 28 (2008): 7911–7918.
6. V. V. Vyazovskiy et al., "Local Sleep in Awake Rats," *Nature* 472 (2011): 443–447.

CHAPTER 6: HOW AND WHY MEMORIES ARE "REPLAYED" IN SLEEP

1. D. Oudiette et al., "Evidence for the Re-enactment of a Recently Learned Behavior during Sleepwalking," *PLoS. One.* 6 (2011): e18056.
2. A. S. Gupta, M. A. van der Meer, D. S. Touretzky, and A. D. Redish, "Hippocampal Replay Is Not a Simple Function of Experience," *Neuron* 65 (2010): 695–705.
3. G. Girardeau, K. Benchenane, S. I. Wiener, G. Buzsaki, and M. B. Zugaro, "Selective Suppression of Hippocampal Ripples Impairs Spatial Memory," *Nat. Neurosci.* 12 (2009): 1222–1223.
4. S. Diekelmann and J. Born, "The Memory Function of Sleep," *Nat. Rev. Neurosci.* 11 (2010): 114–126.
5. G. Tononi and C. Cirelli, "Sleep Function and Synaptic Homeostasis," *Sleep Med. Rev.* 10 (2006): 49–62.

CHAPTER 7: WHAT IS DREAMING AND WHAT DOES IT TELL US ABOUT MEMORY?

1. R. Stickgold, "Sleep-Dependent Memory Consolidation," *Nature* 437 (2005): 1272–1278.
2. W. C. Dement, *Some Must Watch While Some Must Sleep* (New York: W. W. Norton, 1976).
3. J. A. Hobson and R. W. McCarley, "The Brain as a Dream State Generator: An Activation-Synthesis Hypothesis of the Dream Process," *Am. J. Psychiatry* 134 (1977): 1335–1348.
4. M. Solms, "Dreaming and REM Sleep Are Controlled by Different Brain Mechanisms," *Behavioural and Brain Sciences* 23 (2000): 793–1121.
5. D. Foulkes, M. Hollifeld, B. Sullivan, L. Bradley, and R. Terry, "REM Dreaming and Cognitive Skills at Ages 5-8: A Cross Sectional Study," *International Journal of Behavioural Development* 13 (1990): 447–465.
6. R. Levin and R. S. Daly, "Nightmares and Psychotic Decompensation: A Case Study," *Psychiatry* 61 (1998): 217–222.
7. A. Revosuo, "The Reinterpretation of Dreams: An Evolutionary Hypothesis of the Function of Dreaming," *Behavioural Brain Sciences* 23 (2000): 877–901.
8. R. D. Cartwright, "Dreams That Work: The Relation of Dream Incorporation to Adaptation to Stressful Events," *Dreaming* 1, no. 1 (March 1991): 3–9.
9. E. Bokert, "The Effect of Thirst and Related Verbal Stimulus on Dream Reports," *Dissertation Abstracts* 28 (1968): 4753B.
10. K. M. Castellanos, J. A. Hudson, J. Haviland-Jones, and P. J. Wilson, "Does Exposure to Ambient Odors Influence the Emotional Content of Memories?" *Am. J. Psychol.* 123 (2010): 269–279.
11. M. J. Fosse, R. Fosse, J. A. Hobson, and R. J. Stickgold, "Dreaming and Episodic Memory: A Functional Dissociation?" *J. Cogn Neurosci.* 15 (2003): 1–9.
12. T. Nielsen and R. A. Powell, "The Day-residue and Dream-lag Effects: A Literature Review and Limited Replication of Two Temporal Effects in Dream Formation," *Dreaming* (1992): 267–278.
13. E. J. Wamsley, M. Tucker, J. D. Payne, J. A. Benavides, and R. Stickgold, "Dreaming of a Learning Task Is Associated with Enhanced Sleep-dependent Memory Consolidation," *Curr. Biol.* 20 (2010): 850–855.

CHAPTER 8: SLEEP, SEMANTICS, AND THE MIND

1. J. M. Ellenbogen, J. D. Payne, and R. Stickgold, "The Role of Sleep in Declarative Memory Consolidation: Passive, Permissive, Active or None?" *Curr. Opin. Neurobiol.* 16 (2006): 716–722.
2. U. Wagner, S. Gais, H. Haider, R. Verleger, and J. Born, "Sleep Inspires Insight," *Nature* 427 (2004): 352–355.

3. D. J. Cai, S. A. Mednick, E. M. Harrison, J. C. Kanady, and S. C. Mednick, "REM, Not Incubation, Improves Creativity by Priming Associative Networks," *Proc. Natl. Acad. Sci. U.S.A.* 106 (2009): 10130–10134.

4. H. Lau, S. E. Alger, and W. Fishbein, "Relational Memory: A Daytime Nap Facilitates the Abstraction of General Concepts," *PLoS. One.* 6 (2011): e27139.

5. S. J. Durrant, S. A. Cairney, and P. A. Lewis, "Overnight Consolidation Aids the Transfer of Statistical Knowledge from the Medial Temporal Lobe to the Striatum," *Cereb. Cortex* (2012), doi: 10.1093/cercor/bhs244.

6. P. A. Lewis and S. J. Durrant, "Overlapping Memory Replay during Sleep Builds Cognitive Schemata," *Trends Cogn Sci.* 15 (2011): 343–351.

CHAPTER 9: EMOTIONAL MEMORIES AND SLEEP

1. U. Wagner, M. Hallschmid, B. Rasch, and J. Born, "Brief Sleep After Learning Keeps Emotional Memories Alive for Years," *Biol. Psychiatry* 60 (2006): 788–790.

2. C. Johnson and B. Scott, "Eyewitness Testimony and Suspect Identification as a Function of Arousal, Sex of Witness and Scheduling of Interrogation" (paper, American Psychological Association Annual Meeting, Washington, DC, 1976).

3. I. Wilhelm et al., "Sleep Selectively Enhances Memory Expected to Be of Future Relevance," *J. Neurosci.* 31 (2011): 1563–1569.

4. J. M. Saletin, A. N. Goldstein, and M. P. Walker, "The Role of Sleep in Directed Forgetting and Remembering of Human Memories," *Cereb. Cortex* 21 (2011): 2534–2541.

5. S. S. Yoo, N. Gujar, P. Hu, F. A. Jolesz, and M. P. Walker, "The Human Emotional Brain Without Sleep—A Prefrontal Amygdala Disconnect," *Curr. Biol.* 17 (2007): R877–R878.

6. N. Gujar, S. A. McDonald, M. Nishida, and M. P. Walker, "A Role for REM Sleep in Recalibrating the Sensitivity of the Human Brain to Specific Emotions," *Cereb. Cortex* 21 (2011): 115–123.

CHAPTER 10: DOES SLEEP DISARM DANGEROUS EMOTIONS?

1. M. P. Walker and H. E. van der, "Overnight Therapy? The Role of Sleep in Emotional Brain Processing," *Psychol. Bull.* 135 (2009): 731–748.

2. A. R. Damasio, "The Somatic Marker Hypothesis and the Possible Functions of the Prefrontal Cortex," *Philos. Trans. R. Soc. Lond B Biol. Sci.* 351 (1996): 1413–1420.

3. H. E. van der et al., "REM Sleep Depotentiates Amygdala Activity to Previous Emotional Experiences," *Curr. Biol.* 21 (2011): 2029–2032.

4. D. Koren, I. Arnon, P. Lavie, and E. Klein, "Sleep Complaints as Early Predictors of Posttraumatic Stress Disorder: A 1-Year Prospective Study of Injured Survivors of Motor Vehicle Accidents," *Am. J. Psychiatry* 159 (2002): 855–857.

5. T. A. Mellman, V. Bustamante, A. I. Fins, W. R. Pigeon, and B. Nolan, "REM Sleep and the Early Development of Posttraumatic Stress Disorder," *Am. J. Psychiatry* 159 (2002): 1696–1701.

6. K. Nader, G. E. Schafe, and J. E. Le Doux, "Fear Memories Require Protein Synthesis in the Amygdala for Reconsolidation After Retrieval," *Nature* 406 (2000): 722–726.

7. M. P. Walker, T. Brakefield, J. A. Hobson, and R. Stickgold, "Dissociable Stages of Human Memory Consolidation and Reconsolidation," *Nature* 425 (2003): 616–620.

8. B. Rasch, C. Buchel, S. Gais, and J. Born, "Odor Cues During Slow-wave Sleep Prompt Declarative Memory Consolidation," *Science* 315 (2007): 1426–1429.

9. S. Diekelmann, C. Buchel, J. Born, and B. Rasch, "Labile or Stable: Opposing Consequences for Memory When Reactivated During Waking and Sleep," *Nat. Neurosci.* 14, no. 3 (March 2011): 381–386.

10. B. Baran, E. F. Pace-Schott, C. Ericson, and R. M. Spencer, "Processing of Emotional Reactivity and Emotional Memory Over Sleep," *J. Neurosci.* 32 (2012): 1035–1042.

11. K. A. Paller and A. D. Wagner, "Observing the Transformation of Experience into Memory," *Trends Cogn Sci.* 6 (2002): 93–102.

12. H. J. van Marle, E. J. Hermans, S. Qin, S. Overeem, and G. Fernandez, "The Effect of Exogenous Cortisol During Sleep on the Behavioral and Neural Correlates of Emotional Memory Consolidation in Humans," *Psychoneuroendocrinology* (2013), doi: 10.1016/j.psyneuen.2013.01.009.

CHAPTER 11: GOOD SLEEPERS AND BAD SLEEPERS

1. B. A. Mander et al., "Prefrontal Atrophy, Disrupted NREM Slow Waves and Impaired Hippocampal-Dependent Memory in Aging," *Nat. Neurosci.* 16, no. 3 (March 2013): 357–364.

CHAPTER 12: GETTING THE MOST OUT OF YOUR SLEEP

1. L. Marshall, H. Helgadottir, M. Mölle, and J. Born, "Boosting Slow Oscillations During Sleep Potentiates Memory," *Nature* 444 (2006): 610–613.

2. H. V. Ngo, T. Martinetz, J. Born, and M. Mölle, "Auditory Closed-Loop Stimulation of the Sleep Slow Oscillation Enhances Memory," *Neuron,* 78, no. 3 (May 8, 2013): 545–553.

3. B. Rasch, C. Buchel, S. Gais, and J. Born, "Odor Cues During Slow-Wave Sleep Prompt Declarative Memory Consolidation," *Science* 315 (2007): 1426–1429.

4. P. Peigneux et al., "Are Spatial Memories Strengthened in the Human Hippocampus During Slow Wave Sleep?" *Neuron* 44 (2004): 535–545.

5. J. D. Rudoy, J. L. Voss, C. E. Westerberg, and K. A. Paller, "Strengthening Individual Memories by Reactivating Them During Sleep," *Science* 326 (2009): 1079.

6. J. W. Antony, E. W. Gobel, J. K. O'Hare, P. J. Reber, and K. A. Paller, "Cued Memory Reactivation During Sleep Influences Skill Learning," *Nat. Neurosci.* 15 (2012): 1114–1116.

7. D. Bendor and M. A. Wilson, "Biasing the Content of Hippocampal Replay During Sleep," *Nat. Neurosci.* 15 (2012): 1439–1444.

8. A. Arzi, et al. "Humans Can Learn New Information During Sleep," *Nat. Neurosci.* 15 (2012): 1460–1465.

CHAPTER 13: BRIEF NOTES ON HOW TO GET THE SLEEP YOU NEED

1. K. Krauchi, C. Cajochen, E. Werth, and A. Wirz-Justice, "Warm Feet Promote the Rapid Onset of Sleep," *Nature* 401 (1999): 36–37.

2. R. J. Raymann, D. F. Swaab, and E. J. Van Someren, "Cutaneous Warming Promotes Sleep Onset," *Am. J. Physiol Regul. Integr. Comp Physiol* 288 (2005): R1589–R1597.

3. K. M. Sharkey, M. A. Carskadon, M. G. Figueiro, Y. Zhu, and M. S. Rea, "Effects of an Advanced Sleep Schedule and Morning Short Wavelength Light Exposure on Circadian Phase in Young Adults with Late Sleep Schedules," *Sleep Med.* 12 (2011): 685–692.

4. K. Burkhart and J. R. Phelps, "Amber Lenses to Block Blue Light and Improve Sleep: A Randomized Trial," *Chronobiol. Int.* 26 (2009): 1602–1612.

5. M. L. Stanchina, M. bu-Hijleh, B. K. Chaudhry, C. C. Carlisle, and R. P. Millman, "The Influence of White Noise on Sleep in Subjects Exposed to ICU Noise," *Sleep Med.* 6 (2005): 423–428.

6. T. Kawada and S. Suzuki, "Sleep Induction Effects of Steady 60 dB (A) Pink Noise," *Ind. Health* 31 (1993): 35–38.

7. T. Komori, T. Matsumoto, E. Motomura, and T. Shiroyama, "The Sleep-Enhancing Effect of Valerian Inhalation and Sleep-Shortening Effect of Lemon Inhalation," *Chem. Senses* 31 (2006): 731–737; D. M. Taibi, C. A. Landis, H. Petry, and M. V. Vitiello, "A Systematic Review of Valerian as a Sleep Aid: Safe but Not Effective," *Sleep Med. Rev.* 11 (2007): 209–230.

8. M. Schredl et al., "Information Processing During Sleep: The Effect of Olfactory Stimuli on Dream Content and Dream Emotions," *J. Sleep Res.* 18 (2009): 285–290.

index